Asthma and Allergy

solution that works for

COVID-19

The Powerful Natural Prescription for Respiratory Health
During the Coronavirus Pandemic

Dr. Lon Jones, D.O.

Book design by Najdan Mancic

ISBN 978-1-893910-26-3

Freedom Press, Inc.
www.HealthyLivinGMagazine.us
E-mail: info@HealthyLivinGMagazine.us

T his book is dedicated to my mother. Her daily admonishment as she sent me off to school was, "Keep your nose clean." When I got older I asked her whether the reminder was metaphorical or real, and she told me about one of her friends in grammar school who had a chronic runny nose that affected her relationships with her classmates—it wasn't metaphorical. As I learned more about how the body works, it always made sense to try to help our defenses, just like Mom asked me to do. The fact that I finally found a way to honor her request gave her some joy in her final years.

I also dedicate this book to my wife, Jerry Bozeman. She greatly impacted every aspect of what you will read in this book. It was her observation as a special education teacher that there was a connection between chronic ear infections and her students. And when our granddaughter began down that path she said to me, "If somebody really cared about children, they would find a way to prevent ear infections." Having fathered several children of my own as well as being an adoptive, step, and foster father to more, that was a challenge I could not escape. I could not honor her more than did Jerry Klein, the co-author of the standard medical textbook, *Otitis Media in Infants and Children.* "You tell your people," he told us at dinner one time, "that this Jerry agrees with your Jerry." This is in part an explanation of their story as well as mine.

CONTENTS

CHAPTER ONE

A Shift in Focus

As someone who practiced in rural Texas, some consider me a "country doctor"—I've even been called "America's Favorite Country Doctor." I am also an osteopathic physician. While osteopathic physicians and medical doctors study the same material and perform the same function, they go about their job in different ways.

Back in the days when I was looking at medical schools, I wasn't familiar with osteopathic medicine, but I was surprised to see how regular medical schools taught and practiced medicine. The focus seemed to be more on the disease rather than the person. During the time when I considered medical schools, they accepted younger applicants so the graduates could practice longer. With a variety of education and other experiences behind me, I was older and didn't fit that mold. Many MD students were so young they were uncomfortable dealing with people, so they went into specialties like radiology and pathology—specialties where they interacted with patients very little, if at all. I wanted something different. After hearing about osteopathic medicine and doing some research on my own, I knew I had found something more in line with what I wanted.

OSTEOPATHIC MEDICINE VS. ALLOPATHIC WESTERN MEDICINE

Simply put, osteopathic medicine tends to focus more on the person, while traditional western allopathic medicine tends to focus more on the symptoms. One of osteopathic medicine's core principles is that the body can heal itself if it has what it needs and everything is working well. To illustrate this, osteopathic physicians often point to the successful treatment given to Americans suffering from the flu after the World War I pandemic we called the Spanish Flu (though it is thought that the virus actually originated from avian or porcine sources in the American Midwest).

The 1918 flu pandemic killed millions of people around the world. The responsible virus was closely related to the H1N1 flu strain that affected so many persons in 2009. Both are a subtype of the Influenza A virus, which is why people were so concerned back then; the immunity gained a century ago may have worn down.

Now, of course, we face the threat from COVID-19, a novel coronavirus that is ravaging our global population and has killed more than 100,000 Americans alone as I write this. The treatment wisdom that osteopathy had for dealing with the 1918 pandemic has never been so relevant.

In 1919, the people treated in the United States by osteopathic physicians had a mortality rate that was twenty times less than those treated by regular physicians. Originally this was credited to a defining practice of osteopathic medicine called manipulation, a set of techniques using stretching, pressure, and resistance to improve the structure of the body. This is important but misses a key fact—the body is a very complex organism; it's not a machine. For one treatment method to solve many problems is the great exception and certainly not the rule.

In an article in the October 2004 issue of the *Journal of the American Osteopathic Association*, Dr. Harold Magoun, Jr. took another look at why the care given by osteopathic physicians was more successful. He pointed out that the typical practice of regular physicians was to treat a fever with aspirin and the coughing with cough suppressants. Dr. Magoun knew that a fever and a cough are both defenses that help us better cope with invading agents. We have gained those defenses through thousands of years of challenges, and they are indeed the best way—so far—of dealing with them. They are the result of natural selection, and they come with the survival benefit that makes natural selection work. Crippling those defenses meant that those with the flu had less ability to cope with the virus—and more of them died. Osteopathic physicians used neither of these treatments and saw a twentyfold increase in survival because the defenses of the individuals were better able to cope.

When we look at our bodies in the light of our defenses we understand what George Williams and Randolph Nesse talk about in their book, *Why We Get Sick*. A fever is a defense; it handicaps the bacteria and boosts our defenses. Drs. Williams and Nesse point out that artificially infected rabbits die more often when they are treated with the drugs we use to treat a fever. In exactly the same way we handicap ourselves when we treat our other defenses.

WRONG-HEADED FOCUS ON SYMPTOMS

These examples also show one of the major problems in modern medicine—the focus is largely wrong-headed. Western medicine has its roots in "humoral medicine." The Greeks and Romans thought illnesses were caused by an imbalance of the humors—black bile, yellow bile, phlegm, and blood—with each respectively relating to an element, earth, fire, water, and air. Health was defined as a balance of the humors, and treatments were aimed at correcting the imbalance.

For example, when someone showed symptoms of a fever, redness, swelling, or pain, physicians believed there was an imbalance of too much blood. So physicians bled the person until the symptoms got better; bloodletting was the symbol of medicine for more than a thousand years, like the stethoscope is today. And they did get better— if one only looked at the symptoms. If the problem is caused by an injury, like a sprain, for example, the symptoms are indeed related to an excess of blood; the injury triggers the opening of the blood vessels so the area swells to splint the injury, and pain increases so the hurt person doesn't use it. We have learned to treat such injuries by supporting the defenses: we splint the injury and use a sling or crutches so we don't use it. That's wise. These symptoms, like a fever, are a defense. But the loss of blood from the bloodletting is a more critical problem; it trumps all other defenses.

Bloodletting triggers the shock response, which shuts down the blood supply to the extremities, where the sprain is, in order to save more for the critical central organs like the heart, brain, and kidneys. You could literally watch your patient "get better" as the bleeding progressed—the redness, swelling, and pain all disappeared. With this in mind, it is little wonder the practice lasted as long as it did. Bloodletting for injuries was not that harmful, especially if one splinted the injury from the outside as is commonly done, but if it is due to an infection it's a different story.

It wasn't until the middle of the nineteenth century that physicians got around to asking the right question about bloodletting: What does it do to life expectancy in people with pneumonia? They found that more people died after having been bled. In the case of infection, the increased blood supply brings with it a host of defenses to fight the invading bacteria. Blocking that defense gives the edge to the bacteria.

If you ask most physicians about humoral medicine they will likely tell you that they don't practice that way anymore. But the culture of humoral medicine continues today—we have just changed the humors and made them more scientific. The focus remains on symptoms. Our drugs are measured by what they do to the target 'humor' (blood pressure, glucose level, fever), not necessarily what they do to life expectancy.

LEARNING FROM BIOLOGY

One of the things I studied before going to medical school was the history of science and ideas; that's why I was interested in bloodletting. One of the other lessons from that study was the argument between Louis Pasteur and Claude Bernard about the causes of disease. Pasteur argued for the microbe while Bernard spoke of the "soil" where the microbe was planted. In our view today that is basically our ability to cope with the microbe with all of the defenses we have so that we don't get sick. The point that Bernard made was that if our defenses are optimal we can deal with the microbe and not get sick.

Both of these pioneers were correct, but Pasteur gave us something to fight, and threats, like microbes that can kill us, carried the day; so Bernard, even though equally correct, is forgotten. Bernard is known as the father of modern physiology; he needs to be remembered.

Osteopathic physicians seem to share his point of view in their belief that if our structure is optimal we will be healthier, but, unfortunately, most of them have been swallowed up in western medicine with the focus on treating symptoms.

Rather than focus on symptoms, we would be better off learning a lesson from physiologists. They ask why we have symptoms and have found that many are defenses developed through natural selection; that is, they have a significant benefit for survival. Dr. Magoun noted that people have fevers because it helps them deal more effectively with infections—it's a defense that needs to honored and supported rather than just turned off. Biologists overwhelmingly agree. Most physicians understand this too, but they haven't gotten around to looking at the latest studies showing that even with overwhelming infection and high fevers lowering the fever is not helpful.

ADAPTATION AND NATURAL SELECTION

While it is easy to see that some of our symptoms may be defenses, it is harder to see that we adapt; physiologic adaptations are slow and fuzzy, if not invisible. But our view of looking at them changed dramatically after Sir Isaac Newton showed how mechanical the universe was. For almost three centuries the focus of western science has been analytical. When something doesn't work right we take it apart, find what is broken, replace or repair it, and put it back together. That's how early osteopaths saw their patients. In the last three centuries, most of what we have worked with has been mechanical where this method is appropriate. But a human body is not a simple mechanical device; it is not even a complicated mechanical device. The difference is significant, and even some world-class biologists have not seen it. Jacques Monod, a Nobel Prize winning biologist, famously said, "The cell is a machine; the body is a machine; man is a machine." But in this he comes down clearly on the analytical side. Machines can be predicted, but they can't adapt or create something new. Living agents can create novel solutions as they adapt to changes in their environments and these adaptations are not reliably predictable. While there is much in the practice of medicine that is causally related, we would be far better served if medical educators and researchers could see the human body as an adaptive system rather than the mechanical model. This is clearest on a cellular level where there is an ongoing play between our mutating influenza viruses and our own immune adaptations.

My education and experiences have helped me to view the body as a complex and adaptive system. In an earlier book, I talked about how such systems include those we join together to make such as our clubs, states, and nations. They all are complex—having too many variables to calculate or even model—and adaptive—able to create novel solutions that are emergent and unpredictable.

In a way the material here follows this pattern: it is a novel way, because we have forgotten Bernard, a new way of seeing. It started when I began practicing, but it took time to recognize it.

PRIMARY/SECONDARY DEFENSES

We are most vulnerable at our openings—the genitourinary (GU), gastrointestinal (GI), and respiratory tracts; our secondary defenses come into play to help out when the primary defenses are not up to the task.

Primary defenses work all the time and don't have any associated symptoms. We take them for granted most of the time. They work in the background as quietly as antivirus software on your computer.

Secondary defenses have symptoms, so that we know something is wrong, and our body needs help. Mostly these secondary defenses include washing and cleansing actions such as leukorrhea (a purulent discharge in the GU tract); nausea, vomiting, and diarrhea for the gut; and rhinorrhea (a runny nose) for the respiratory tract.

ORAL REHYDRATION THERAPY

I began practicing in 1974, and one of the things I read about then was the use of oral rehydration therapy (ORT) in treating cholera. One editorial comment was that ORT had saved more lives in ten years than penicillin did in forty. I was impressed, especially since it was something everyone could mix up at home. In 1974, the costs of health care were still manageable, but the trajectory was concerning; I liked things that could be made at home. How to make and use ORT at home became one of the most useful prescriptions that I handed out in my practice.

Clinical therapy with ORT had been researched in the 1960s, but without a drug classification there was no money behind it. But with cholera epidemics killing millions in third-world countries its need was clear, and studies were done. It works because it triggers the sodium-glucose transport system in the stomach, which has been measured at the molecular level, so we know that two molecules of the salt (sodium), one molecule of sugar (glucose), and 264 molecules of water are pumped into the body from the stomach. Using ORT, although basic, is the most effective, efficient, and safest way to get water into the body. It took a while to realize that its success was because it optimized our natural GI defenses by simply keeping the body's tank of water full. This allowed the GI tract to perform its immune functions and begin to attack the causative agent while it was still in the stomach.

Learning takes time. I can't say I learned all this quickly. A lot of it was adaptive, trying to help patients or at home with family. In fact, it wasn't until far into this story that I actually realized how everything fit together in what I call defense medicine. But these treatments don't make any money for the industry. None of the methods used to help our defenses are drugs. That's bad news for the drug industry, but it's good news for you. If your defensive team is optimal you don't need much of an offense, and it's the same with our bodies.

WOMEN'S GENITOURINARY DEFENSES

Although my primary focus in this book is on respiratory health, I would be remiss if I didn't discuss support for women's defenses. This is especially important because the same concept of biofilms and bacterial populations, components of what we call our mucosal immune system, apply to all three areas.

Your GI, GU, and respiratory tracts are almost entirely made up of friendly biofilm; in both sexes, this includes biofilm that lines the urethra and the vagina in women. Regular washing with urination and menstruation helps and is more natural and less disruptive than douching.

Before we realized this, however, the standard treatment that many doctors advocated was douching, aimed at washing out the irritant. But this also washed out the friendly bacteria and opened the area to other more infectious bacteria. Studies demonstrated this, and the practice was stopped. Now more treatments are aimed at making sure this biofilm is populated with friendly Lactobacilli bacterial strains.

While I didn't have the connection then, when Jerry pointed to our granddaughter's chronic, painful ear infections that left her wailing and suggested in her kind yet demanding way that I do something different I knew what I had to do: find out why our granddaughter's nasal defenses were crippled and how to fix them.

The largest percentage of my patients had respiratory problems, from allergies and asthma, to ear and sinus infections, with colds and the flu always prevalent. All of these are connected to the nose, which is where they start. My experience is not unique. Studies show that upper respiratory problems are the number one reason for visiting your doctor.

You would think that things might be different living in the middle of the largest of the lower states where we are free from urban pollution. But even here in the bare lands of Texas we have enough pollution from agricultural use of fertilizers, aerial pesticide spraying, and dust storms (to say nothing of the dust from cotton gins during harvest season) to have many of the same problems that occur in highly urbanized and industrialized regions. It is also hot and dry, which leads to other issues that handicap our health. In any event, upper respiratory problems are a major problem in the health of our people, just as they are in the rest of the nation. Because of the stories I am going to relate, I came to be known as the go-to doctor when it comes to upper respiratory problems. Patients often came to me after they or their children were prescribed multiple drugs or received surgery for their problem. Luckily, I had a better, natural solution to help them: a nasal spray that strengthens and enhances our normal nasal defenses. It is very simple and safe, and has been proven effective in studies throughout the world. It honors what my Mom told me every day: "Keep your nose clean!" She couldn't have been more right.

In fact, as you will come to see, the same principles we will learn about in the rest of this book are quite applicable to self-protection when it comes to COVID-19.

This book is not about osteopaths or osteopathic medicine, although that founding principle is in every page. It is about how we can help our defenses, particularly those in the nose, and how optimizing those defenses can virtually eliminate upper respiratory problems including COVID-19. This is the primary message, but it needs to be in the context of "Defense Medicine," which is aimed at preventing illnesses in all areas.

Now, let me tell you about some of my own case histories that helped me to gather the medical knowledge to help you now during these troubling times.

CASE 1

Heather, our granddaughter, suffered from recurring ear infections. She was the reason for the development of the first-generation spray that I came to develop. Heather was breast fed until she was two years old and neither parent smoked, so she had little risk for ear infections. But when she was five-months old, her parents placed her in day care so that her mother could return to teaching school. Within two months she had an ear infection. It was treated and resolved with antibiotics, but the infections returned. Within five months she'd had four more.

That's when Jerry panicked and dropped the challenge that if I really cared about kids I would find a solution. The idea was prompted by a report in the *British Medical Journal* by Matti Uhari, a Finnish pediatric infectious-disease doctor. Dr. Uhari showed that chewing xylitol-sweetened gum five times a day significantly reduced ear infections. In Finland, the government provides this gum for children in school because it prevents tooth decay. When I told Jerry about the gum she just said, "By the time she's old enough to chew gum she'll be deaf."

Since the germs causing ear infections start in the nose, we decided to put it there in small amounts.

Xylitol is a food—it's a sugar substitute and plentiful in many fruits such as apples and plums. It isn't absorbed in the nose, and a person could use it every hour, twenty-four hours a day, both sides of the nose, and get about half a plum's worth of xylitol. We figured it was safe, and the Food and Drug Administration (FDA) agreed. This is how it all started.

Heather's parents and day care workers understood the need for consistency when using the spray. They cooperated in spraying her nose every time they changed her diaper. Once she began using the nasal spray, she had no further ear infections until about six months later when a new daycare worker was hired who was not aware of the spraying routine. Reestablishing regular nasal washing resolved this problem without the need for antibiotics. She continues to use this spray on a regular basis and averaged less than one fever a year throughout her four years in day care—far less than the normal six upper respiratory infections (URIs) per year for children attending day care. Her only antibiotic use since has been when she had a sore throat and tested positive for strep.

CASE 2

Traci was nine and suffered from asthma so badly she was in the emergency room at least once a month. She was on five different medications for her asthma including systemic steroids that are known to block growth.

Traci's mother wanted to know if the nasal spray my wife and I had recently developed would help her daughter. I told her it wouldn't hurt to try. Her mother gave Traci the xylitol-based nasal spray four times a day and continued giving her the other medications. About a week later, her mom was washing Traci's hair when Traci began gagging, choking, coughing, and wound up vomiting.

Traci got rid of a bunch of thick, jelly-like tissue. Her mom thought she was losing her brains. A week later though, Traci noticed that she didn't have any problem breathing. Two weeks later she continued to breathe quite easily, so her mom and I decided to gradually stop her asthma medications. Still no problems. Six months later, Traci was playing basketball and doing gymnastics with no wheezing at all. But what does washing your nose have to do with asthma? Well, that's what I'm going to explore with you a bit later.

CASES 3-12

After Heather's story appeared in a local paper, I soon had many other similar children in my practice coming from all over the place. I only saw these children a few times usually, so this is certainly not a double-blind, placebo-controlled, randomized, and peer-reviewed study on resolving ear infections, but I was able to later get follow-up information on how ten of these kids did. In the five months before I saw them, they had been taken to the doctor and received antibiotics for ear complaints a total of forty-three times. Over the average of eleven months that we watched these children and their noses were washed just like Heather's, they went to the doctor for ear complaints and received antibiotics a total of seven times. That's more than a 94-percent reduction in doctor visits and antibiotic use. The results could've been better because of the seven times they went to the doctor, three were in one child, and three occurred when the parents had run out of the spray. Those extra three would have made it 95 percent. This was certainly not the standard, controlled study FDA requires for efficacy, but recent trends have shown that parental reporting of ear complaints in their children is often as reliable as a doctor's exam.

Since all URIs follow essentially the same pattern, with the virus or bacteria first colonizing the nose and then spreading to other areas to trigger infections, results like these are the basis of our hope to eliminate upper respiratory problems. And it is not just children who benefit.

CASE 13

Beth was an elementary school teacher. Her extensive close contact with children heightened the risk of getting lots of sinus infections. By the time she came to me, she had almost given up on the medical profession because the continuous use of antibiotics didn't seem to help. She even got to the point where she would wear a bandanna tucked behind her glasses to catch the sinus drainage when she bent over to help her students. After she started using the spray regularly, her problem significantly decreased, but she still had occasional episodes where she relied on her topical decongestants to help open her nose. For reasons that we will discuss later I don't think that is a good idea. Instead, I encouraged Beth to lie down for a few minutes on her back, put a few drops of our spray in each nostril, and wait a few minutes to allow the solution to get to the back of the nose. This seemed to do the trick and Beth has been free of problems ever since.

CASE 14

DC, 42, had diabetes and asthma for about twenty years. She was on multiple medications for her asthma, including steroids that made her diabetes harder to manage. She went to the hospital for her asthma and related pulmonary infections an average of two times annually for ten years. She began using the xylitol nasal spray regularly and in the ensuing year did not experience any asthma and did not require any asthma medication. After such a long time with asthma, DC's airway had narrowed, decreasing the amount of air able to pass through it. Doctors dealing with chronic asthma argue that this remodeling is permanent. Peak flow is the amount of air the person can move as they breathe; it reflects the size of the airway. DC's peak flow remained at 150 to 200 for about six months, which wasn't very good and reflected her remodeled airways. But after a year of regularly cleaning her nose, it increased to 350.

CASE 15

Jim worked at the local meat-packing plant in the warehouse. He drove a forklift and was in and out of the freezer all day long. The constant temperature change wreaked havoc with his sinuses. He'd used a nasal decongestant for years, which enabled him to breathe easier but seemed to make his nose worse. Within a week after using of the xylitol spray he had "a new life."

These cases are just a few of thousands who have seen their upper respiratory problems—including middle-ear infections, allergies, asthma and sinus infections—disappear when they began their nasal hygiene program. The spray doesn't do anything to the viruses or irritants that trigger our infections or allergies or asthma; it is not an offensive weapon like antibiotics. All it does is support our defensive team.

As we should have learned earlier from our experience with the 1918 flu pandemic, strengthening our defensive team will help to win the game everyone is playing with the infectious and noxious elements in our environment. To be sure, not everyone is cured so easily; some seem to get no benefit. We feel sure that getting to these people earlier, while their defenses are still intact, would enable them also to realize the benefits that thousands of others have experienced.

THE OFFENSIVE VS. DEFENSE APPROACH

Like any sports team, our defenses need to be strongest where we are most vulnerable, and our bodies are most vulnerable at our openings. Our noses are the opening to the respiratory tract. Almost all URIs begin here, where all of the pollutants and germs we breathe enter the body and the respiratory tract begins. Most URIs are the result of viral infections, opening the doors for bacteria to infect the body further and vice versa; it's as if they intuitively and instinctively cooperate, knowing their biological interests in recycling us are shared.

Colds and flu happen all year long, but in the temperate zones of the world they are much more concentrated in the fall and winter months—we call this cold and flu season. There is not a flu season in the tropics—a fact I will explain later. While colds and flu impact everyone, they are more of a problem for the very young and the very old where they kill more often.

As the examples above suggest, I also feel safe in saying that the vast majority, if not all, of these infections are unnecessary. In dealing with these infecting problems in the past, we have concentrated our efforts on relieving symptoms or stopping the infectious agent. We have developed antibiotics that kill them or immunizations that help our bodies resist and kill them. We concentrate on the offensive aspects of this warfare and ignore the defenses we all have that help us to survive in the midst of our polluted and bacteria-laden world. Indeed with the wonders of modern medicine we are more likely to hobble our defenses than help them.

We do this because that is how we think about our problems in medicine. Five-hundred years ago, people thought sinning or some other wrongful action caused illness, which was punishment from the gods. But some 350 years ago a British physician named Thomas Sydenham turned this theory upside down. He lived during the last of the bubonic plagues and saw many different people that shared similar patterns in their illnesses. He thought illnesses came from something outside the body other than the gods, and his view came to be accepted over the years. It was given a tremendous boost when Louis Pasteur showed how anthrax was caused by a bacterium and proposed the germ theory of disease—germs from outside us caused disease. To repeat what I said earlier, Pasteur gave us something to fight. Threats like this send us to what is descriptively called our fight, or flight response where the options for action are limited to fight, flight, or freeze. These responses are tactical. Strategy needs a safe place to think that isn't there in the presence of a threat.

If you haven't noticed this is true for our nation as well as all of us. This viewpoint continues to spread as we find infections associated with ulcers, heart disease, even cervical and breast cancer. So we have concentrated our efforts on finding and eliminating these external agents. We have concentrated on the offensive, on finding ways to kill or incapacitate the opposition.

Economist James K. Galbraith coined the term "conventional wisdom" to describe how a society comes to share a concept or viewpoint, which is always fostered by profit. So, too, in the conventional wisdom of medicine, the focus on the offensive is strongly influenced by profits.

MEDICAL CARE'S MOTIVES: PROFIT OR BETTER HEALTH?

Learning about ORT had an early impact on my thinking in medical practice. We would likely not know as much about oral rehydration were it not for a charitable non-governmental organization in Bangladesh where people knew the research and had a continual problem with cholera. Cholera kills, not because of the infection per se, but because the body tries to wash out the toxins so vigorously that it loses fluid too rapidly to replace. While cholera gets the blame, the cause of death is typically dehydration.

Hundreds of Bangladeshi women were trained to educate the people about oral rehydration and the simple solution: a glass of water, a fist full of sugar, and a pinch of salt—and drink more than you lose. Thousands of lives were saved because of this simple treatment, and the editors of the British medical journal *Lancet* called this episode in health one of the greatest achievements of twentieth-century medicine. It is by far the most effective and efficient way of getting water into the body that we have. But few people in this country know about it, a situation that leaders at Johns Hopkins called lamentable.

The reasons that so few know about oral rehydration are several: first of all, salt and sugar are not patentable, so this mixture cannot be a drug, even though it treats an illness effectively and saves thousands of lives. No drug status means no drug claims and no advertising; and in our society that translates to no one knowing. The second reason is our health-care system's position on profits. If a person has the stomach flu and goes to the local emergency room, treatment will be with an IV, which increases both the level of care and the complexity of the service so the hospital can bill in the highest range of profit; this is even though a bottle of Pedialyte® would likely have been as good in resolving the problem.

The story and the success of oral rehydration convinced me that there may be other cures out there just waiting to be found that are equally effective. As it turns out the reason both oral rehydration and the nasal spray we developed are so medically successful is that both support a defense.

However, they are not well known because they are not drugs.

The profit-oriented viewpoint, when it dominates our view and controls the narrative as it does today in medicine, blinds us to seeing the many defenses that protect us from invading pollutants. It feeds off our offensive focus, and we now know that focus leads to resistance in the microbes as they learn how to cope and share that learning with any other microbe that needs it. This is a war we cannot win. On the other hand, we know how our defenses work, and we know that they act in ways that don't trigger defenses in the microbes. The end result of this is that our warfare leads to increased virulence in the microbes, while helping our defenses leads to less virulence and more friendly bacteria. This is the idea behind Paul Ewald's book, *Evolution of Infectious Disease*.

In this book, we are going to focus on the respiratory tract, the source of URIs, allergies, asthma, and where COVID-19 stages its horrendous attacks on the human body, and all of the other problems that begin in the back of the nose. We will also delve into lower-respiratory infections as well since most pulmonary infections, like pneumonia and bronchitis, begin with bacteria that first colonize the nose. These microbes hold on to cells in our noses and multiply. They break off as biofilms (much like plaque in our arteries) and are aspirated into the lungs to cause problems there. Other lung diseases, like pulmonary fibrosis, originate in response to irritants that escape our nasal defenses and get into the lungs.

Along with the trachea that goes to the lungs, there are openings in the upper part of the nose that lead to our sinuses; the Eustachian canal goes to the middle ear, and there are tear ducts leading to the eyes. All of these connected areas commonly get infected from bacteria living in the back of the nose. Honoring and supporting our nasal defenses means diminishing problems because the irritants and infecting agents will not be there.

Washing your nose with a simple spray will help you to overcome allergies, asthma, sinus problems, middle ear infections, and even help your body to cope better with whatever bugs are in the air during cold and flu season. That's our argument in a nutshell: Keep your nose clean and you can get rid of these problems for good.

CHAPTER TWO

The Discovery: Ear Infections and Human Development

My wife Jerry was trained in special education and much of her teaching career has been working with children who are not able to learn using traditional methods. Early on, she recognized that many of her students with language learning problems had a history of chronic ear infections when they were young (before age two). This became clear when talking to parents at the annual review meetings and when she asked her students, "Did you have tubes put in your ears when you were young?" Most of the time the answer was, "Yes." While Jerry knew there was a connection she didn't know why.

When ear infections become chronic, fluid produced by the body (an attempt to wash away infection) stays in the middle ear—the shaded area in the image. The longer it stays there the thicker it gets—the Brits call it "glue ear," as shown in Figure 2.1 (next page). The middle ear is home to all of the small bones that carry the vibrations of the eardrum to the brain. The "glue" eliminates that transmission so the pathways in the brain are not used. At about age two, a process takes place in the brain that removes many of the unused pathways. This pruning coincides with the end of the developmental window for learning language. These windows are periods of time when the brain is set up for learning in specific areas, and when the window closes learning is much harder. This is how persistent inner-ear fluid becomes a brain problem and why special education has grown so much in line with the increases in ear infections.

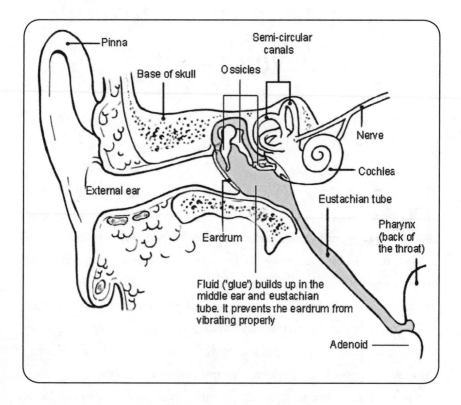

Figure 2.1 *Glue Ear*

Dr. Jerry Klein is the author of the textbook *Otitis Media in Infants and Children*. In the past, ear infections (otitis media is the technical term) were considered something kids just had to go through, like a rite of passage. There was little to no discussion of the learning problems. That ended when later editions of the textbook addressed these problems.

Tubes are inserted into a child's eardrum with recurring ear infections in the attempt to reduce the fluid in the middle ear. This procedure is designed to help with hearing by allowing the fluid to drain, but it doesn't reduce the frequency of infections. Indeed, by putting a hole in the ear drum it opens the middle ear to the outside environment. Language, a critical part of early learning, is built through day-to-day hearing during the developmental window—the same period when ear infections are most common. If the hearing is dampened by infection or fluid in the middle ear during this important period, it takes persistent and determined effort on the part of parents and teachers to overcome the deficit.

Dr. M. Luotonen and co-researchers demonstrated in the October 1996 issue of *Pediatric Infectious Disease Journal* that, even when properly treated, recurrent ear infections during the first two years result in significant impairment in reading ability up to the age of nine. Dr. K.E. Bennett and co-researchers reported in the August 2001 issue of *Archives of Diseases in Children* that they followed the children longer and found significant learning and social problems extending up to age eighteen.

There are also now conditions like post-otitis auditory disorder (POAD) or central auditory processing dysfunction (CAPD) that reflect and recognize some of the long-term problems associated with chronic ear infections. However, most physicians have not made a connection; they see these as educational problems, not medical. These long-term studies show that tubes don't help much to reduce the educational problems that accompany chronic ear infections. If the problem is not dealt with, the child can get frustrated with the educational process and often develops behavioral problems.

There is not much that medicine can do when these infections become chronic. In fact, the United Kingdom's National Health Service no longer treats patients with the condition. Doctors just give them pain medicine and wait for it to resolve on its own. Many doctors turn to antibiotics, which don't seem to help much. Despite the ineffectiveness, we in the United States often wait several months for a trial of antibiotics before placing the tubes without even considering that this period of time eliminates even more of this crucial developmental window. While POAD and CAPD are known, they have not made it into our standard list of medical conditions and continue to be ignored by the medical profession. These long-term educational handicaps rob our children of optimal growth and development.

As physicians we tend to ignore this problem of fluid in the middle ear, thinking that if there is no infection the fluid eventually will go away. In the meantime it contributes substantially to the population of children in our special education programs and to the expense that goes along with them. This educational expense is not even considered in the figures showing the costs of ear infections, but ear infections are one of the most common causes of special education services—and they are preventable. Jerry wouldn't let me ignore it. We need to realize that the billions of dollars we could save by preventing ear infections is only a fraction of their cost to our educational systems.

EARLY STEPS

Three months after Heather's condition resolved and her symptoms had disappeared, her dad suggested that I get the spray patented, which I did. I also went to the FDA and told them I had a way to wash the nose. The FDA responded that they did not have a category for a nose wash and asked what cleaning the nose did. When I told them of my observations, they said it was a drug.

Drugs are substances that prevent, treat, or improve a medical condition, and the xylitol saline spray certainly fit. However, a hundred years ago when the FDA was started, there were arguments whether to include soap because it does this as well. In fact, the Centers for Disease Control and Prevention (CDC) tells us how important it is to wash our hands to prevent the spread of infection, especially now during this time of coronavirus. But the soap industry didn't want government control, so cleaning the body was left out of the FDA's purview despite its "drug" benefit in preventing illnesses. I tried going through the FDA, but it soon became clear that I didn't have the money or backing to pay for the process. New drugs at that time usually cost at least a million dollars. And if I did borrow that money I would have to charge so much for the "drug" that people would go to the store to buy xylitol and make it themselves. I went to the pharmaceutical industry, but their initial interest evaporated for the same reason.

I contacted a lawyer familiar with FDA issues, and he suggested selling "soap for the nose." Indeed, we encouraged its frequent use just like soap and water.

The patent I got was a "use" patent, meaning that no one could market the nasal use of xylitol. Drug companies want a patent either on the active ingredient, the drug itself, or on the medical device that delivers it. This is the problem we share with oral rehydration; both have sufficient benefit to be classified as "drugs," but neither have the ability to reward the drug companies with sufficient profits to make FDA approval practical. Again: no patent—no profits; no profits— no research; no research—no FDA approval; no FDA approval—no advertising; and, no advertising—no one believes you have anything worthwhile. There is no economical way that a common, safe food substance can be a "drug," so this spray is not regulated or approved by the FDA. It is not a drug; in the eyes of the regulatory authorities, it is only a very neat way to keep your nose clean. If washing your hands is effective in reducing communicable diseases, washing the nose is even more so because that is where so many of them enter the body.

Yet research done on nasally administered xylitol satisfies the most demanding standards: it acts locally and is not absorbed into the nasal tissues. That means that it winds up in our stomachs just like the xylitol we eat in berries or other fruits.

A year after the successful treatment for Heather, the local paper ran a story on what happened, and you know the subsequent story from there. I also treated a second child, JM, with the xylitol saline spray. His mother was also a special-education teacher. JM had already had two sets of ventilation tubes in his ears. After the second set came out, the eardrum did not heal so he needed surgery for repair. Even after these measures, he still had a condition called chronic suppurative otitis media, which is persistent fluid in the middle ear not associated with infection. This is the type of problem that eventually goes away as the child gets older. JM took longer and kept having problems. There is no treatment for this condition except waiting or putting in another set of tubes, but as noted above there are findings now that tubes do not really help the hearing and language problems that accompany the fluid associated with the condition.

JM's mother sprayed his nose without fail. Three days after starting, he gagged and vomited a huge amount of mucus. From that time on he was better. The volume on the TV went down. He was better at discriminating word sounds, and the dark areas under his eyes went away. Two weeks later his auditory test for how well his eardrums were functioning, known a tympanogram, was normal.

From these initial experiences, I knew that xylitol was something special, and believed it had great potential to help in so many other ways as well.

WHAT IS XYLITOL?

Technically xylitol is the sugar alcohol of xylose, which is wood sugar. But that is misleading because xylitol is neither a sugar, nor an alcohol. It looks like sugar and it tastes like sugar, but it has very little effect on a person's blood sugar and is metabolized in an entirely separate way from the other sugars we eat.

Xylose, wood sugar, is actually a very common sugar in the human body. It is one of several sugars that are on our cell surfaces that enable other cells to recognize one another. It is by means of this system of sugars that our cells hold on to each other. It is also these same sugar complexes that bacteria attach to. Most of the sugars we use for energy have a chemical makeup consisting of six carbon atoms. Glucose and fructose are examples of six-carbon sugars. Some of these sugars have unfamiliar names like galactose, mannose, and fucose. Xylose and xylitol only have five carbons. Xylitol also differs from the others in that it is a flexible compound. In the body, the six-carbon sugars are generally fixed in their shape; they are in a ring form that can bind easily and regularly with other sugars to form chains of simple sugars. They are stable enough that other cells and bacteria looking for something to hold on to can rely on them. Xylose is also commonly in a ring formation, but xylitol is only open. This means that it is flexible—it can bend and twist and look like a lot of these other receptors. In other words, it can fill up the connectors, called lectins, the bacteria use to hold on. This is significant to how xylitol works. Despite xylitol's seeming simplicity, it is actually quite a sophisticated method of defensive medicine.

Another reason xylitol works is suggested from the early dental studies; in effect, xylitol gives the bacteria indigestion—they eat it, but they can't digest it. Was this happening in the nose too? I called my colleague Dr. Matti Uhari, a pioneer in xylitol research and author of the chewing-gum study that started me on this track, and told him of my experience. He told me about a study his group had performed that was as yet unpublished. In this study they showed that xylitol blocked much of the bacteria's ability to hold on to the cells in our noses. We will also talk more about this study a little later, but it is a major part of this story because it shows that the action is not just bacterial indigestion.

NASAL CONNECTION

Keeping the nose clean with xylitol is important because essentially all respiratory problems begin there. With its connections to the ears, sinuses, eyes and lungs it acts as a nidus, a nest from which bacteria and viruses spread to other parts of the body. All of these interconnected areas can get irritated by allergens or infected by viruses or bacteria that live in the back of the nose. Honoring and supporting our nasal defenses in their attempts to wash out these irritants results in reduced problems.

TAMING ALLERGIES

The first person who used the xylitol nasal spray for allergies was my grandson Joe, who was allergic to grandmother's cat, when he and his parents were due for a visit. My daughter called and asked what to do. I gave her all of the normal things to do to avoid exposure: shampoo the carpets, keep the cat outside, reserve a close motel room in case, and stock up on antihistamines. I also sent her a bottle of the spray. She used it about every four hours, and Joe had no problems except when he first woke up after a night's rest when mom noticed some swelling around the eyes. This was gone about thirty minutes after the first spray. Dad took the kids back for another visit several months later and was there for about four hours when Joe's face started swelling. He called my daughter and asked her to send the spray. After a night elsewhere they were able to resume the visit with regular use of the spray.

OVERCOMING ASTHMA

Joe, like many other children with allergies, has developed asthma and has an inhaler at home for bronchodilator treatments. He has begun washing his nose regularly and finds that three times a day, with more on occasion when he gets challenged, is enough to keep him clear with no asthma symptoms. Happily, he is able to avoid the drug treatment.

Asthma is such a difficult disease. Seldom is a condition associated with such a profound and anxiety-producing threat as shutting down one's ability to breathe. But the drugs we use to treat it can be a problem too. Admittedly, they are not as toxic as they used to be. In years past we did not have a treatment that could relax constricting airway muscles without speeding up the heart rate. In those days, it seemed that almost as many people died from over-dosing as from asthma; I even had a classmate in medical school that died from asthma drugs. Unfortunately, more and more asthma cases are being reported throughout the country, especially in urban areas, but also where there is a lot of agriculture. However, by washing the nose of contaminants that cause asthma with the xylitol saline spray, asthmatic episodes decrease.

THE SINUS LINK

Sinus infections are similar to ear infections, and both Jerry and I used to have recurring sinus infections. I had used saline off and on for twenty years previous to my discovery and found that it reduced the frequency of my infections a little. I began washing my nose with the xylitol, and Jerry used saline. We were away at a conference when she got her last sinus infection—she was not happy being the control in our two-person study. Now she is using the xylitol spray, and we have both been free of any further sinus infections!

That result was the same found by Dr. Talal Nsouli, the Washington, D.C. doctor who treated President Bill Clinton for his allergies. Dr. Nsouli thought that using a neti pot to wash the nose was similar to the douching we discussed earlier and harmful to the friendly bacteria that even in the nose offer some protection. He did a study, reporting it at a conference of allergists and immunologists, showing an increase in sinus problems in those using a neti pot regularly. Then some of his patients told him about our xylitol spray and how well it worked for them. So he did another study. He had some of his patients use it just three times a day, which was enough to clear most sinus infections in two weeks. When this information was presented at the 2015 conference of the American College of Allergy, Asthma, and Immunology the only question was, "Why not more often?" I totally agree.

The question you have is probably the same one I had: How can one simple spray help with so many diverse health issues?

Again, the answer has to do with our defenses. Our body's defenses are the best available and concentrated where they can do the most good—in the areas of our bodies that are open the environment. In this case, respiratory health begins with your nose.

CHAPTER THREE

Your Nose and Your Defenses

Upper-respiratory infections and conditions are the most common complaints primary-care physicians deal with, and they all start in the back of the nose. This may be repetitious, but it's important. Beginning from their home in the back of the nose, bacteria move down the eustachian canal to cause ear infections, mostly in children. They also climb up into the sinuses, causing infections, mostly in older people. While properly termed lower-respiratory infections, some airborne bacteria and viruses avoid capture by our nasal defenses and are breathed into the lungs, causing bronchitis and pneumonia, but most of them are found in our noses, too.

The major pathogen in the nose, *Streptococcus pneumoniae*, is responsible for the deaths of about 40,000 Americans every year and over a million cases of mortality worldwide, but this particular bacteria, and its family, turns out to be particularly susceptible to xylitol. This was the study that Dr. Uhari told me about as related in Chapter Two.

His team was able to show in the January 2001 issue of the journal *Antimicrobial Agents and Chemotherapy:* ". . . that xylitol is the only commercially used sugar substitute proven to have an antimicrobial effect on pneumococci."

Upper respiratory conditions are a major cause of loss time at work and they have many associated problems even after we recover from the illness. Furthermore the treatment of these conditions is the primary reason for the use of antibiotics, often even when antibiotics are not going to be very helpful. To go along with that, the over-utilization of these antibiotics promotes antibiotic resistance. Upper-respiratory conditions are a major problem, for the illnesses they cause, the effects of those illnesses, and the super bugs that are the bacterial species' reaction to our antibiotics. And the problem is likely to worsen.

Doctors often turn to antibiotics because they kill the invading organism, and most of the time the person suffering gets better. But we know now that antibiotics don't do much when these infections become chronic. We also know that the bacteria in our gut are often killed as well, and they are the ones that help us digest our food, make vitamins and other substances that we need in order to live, and are part of our primary gastrointestinal defense system. And when antibiotics threaten these GI bacteria, they develop resistance as well.

Every living organism has some ability to read its environment and adapt to it, but few do it as speedily as bacteria. We know, for example, that bacteria increase their mutation rate when they are threatened. If enough of them participate in this mutation, a solution to the threat is not far off. These bacteria share the successful mutation with neighboring bacteria that are interested, even those unrelated. So now we have antibiotic-resistant bacteria out in our communities and around the world.

So far our response to this threat has been to rely on ever more powerful antibiotics; that's what you do in a war. We kill more bacteria, but also stimulate more resistance. We are engaged in an arms race with bacteria, a race that for several reasons we have little chance of winning.

UNWINNABLE ARMS RACE

First, bacteria are the most persisting of species by any measure. Humans have existed on earth for less than three-hundred thousand years. Bacteria have existed for four-billion years, and for the first three billion they were the only show in town. They win by measures such as length of dominion, prospects for survival, tenacity, sheer abundance, genetic or biochemical diversity, and range of current habitats. Dr. Stephen Gould, the evolutionary biologist, calls them the titans of life on earth.

The rules in the arms race are also different and handicap our side. In order to develop a new antibiotic, the following elements are necessary: a patent to insure that the company can make a profit; lots of expensive research (they need to test on animals first, and because of this, some of the new antibiotics already have bacteria resistant to them by the time they are released for human use); and they need patients or insurance companies who can pay for them to support more research. This process takes years.

On the other hand, the development of resistance in bacteria is much faster. Most resistance comes from bacteria living in biofilms. We will talk a lot more about biofilms later on, but they are essentially homes for the germs that protect them from antibiotics. It takes about 100-times the normal dose of antibiotics to penetrate into these homes and that much is often toxic to the patient. These bacteria don't get the full dose, but they still see the threat and can increase their mutation rate by more than 1000 times. Not all of them do this because if they all started mutating it would be suicidal. Mutation is a random process and leads to more problems than successes, but there are enough bacteria mutating that resistance comes relatively rapidly. The resistant mutation is multiplied when the bacterium divides, and it is shared with other bacteria with none of our interest in profiting or intellectual property rights. They win both in speed and variety.

A realistic look at the past shows us our odds in this warfare. Bacteria were the first forms of life on our planet. For about three billion years they were the only life. They formed the atmosphere we breathe. They learned to recycle themselves and whatever else they could digest. Some of them learned to use the energy from sunlight and others learned to make it from sugars. About a billion-and-a-half-years ago some of these bacteria cooperated and gave up their individual lives to be a part of a larger cell. The bacteria that knew how to make energy from sugars became the mitochondria that supply the energy for all cells, and the bacteria that had learned how to use sunlight became the chloroplasts that are in all plant cells. Millions of different life forms came from that cooperative beginning, but now, a billion and a half years later, more than 95 percent of these advanced life forms are extinct. On the other hand, 99 percent of the bacteria living at that time are still around. Those are not very good odds when one is choosing sides in a war.

In a dramatic sense, this is a "cosmic war," a battle between the forces of good and those of evil, and the only way to win a cosmic war, according to Iranian-American scholar of religious studies Reza Aslan in his book *How to Win a Cosmic War*, is not to fight one. In our warfare with bacteria this means, as countless specialists have repeatedly pointed out, we need to control our use of antibiotics. But many scientists and medical professionals don't know what to do instead. Keeping your nose clean with xylitol is a first step!

A COUNTRY DOCTOR'S VIEW

Not only does our health-care system not have a workable plan to deal with antibiotic resistance, but the incidence of upper respiratory problems has increased over the past forty years. Some feel that part of the reason for this is how our system works. In a provocative article entitled "Is U.S. Health Really the Best in the World?" published in the July 26, 2000, issue of *The Journal of the American Medical Association,* Barbara Starfield, MD, MPH, offers facts that show that our health-care system is the third leading cause of death in this country behind only heart disease and cancer. To come to this conclusion, she looked mostly at our hospital infections, our surgical errors, and the complications of our drugs. She did not, however, look at the effect of our drugs in turning off many of our more uncomfortable defenses as discussed earlier. Though it was not considered a problem, it still makes our health-care system even more dangerous. For example, she did not look at the recent withdrawal of cold and cough medicines for children, which came as a result of finding that several kids had died following the use of these readily available drugs. While the FDA and pharmaceutical industry blame parents for the overuse of drugs, which compounded their side effects, no one sees the simple connection that these drugs block a helpful defense, eliminating its survival benefit. Eliminating a survival benefit means more people will die, and that is what happened.

There is also an interesting correlation between the use of these drugs and an increase in upper respiratory problems. Side-effect studies for these drugs are done before the FDA will allow them to be released, but the studies look only at the side effects for taking the drug, like sedation, sleep disturbance, nausea, or dry nose, for antihistamines. Few of them ask the question that really matters: what the drug does to long-term health and life expectancy? The studies usually last about two weeks, which is normally long enough to see the side effects, but nowhere near long enough to see the long-term results of taking the drugs. In the case of the cough and cold pills, it took about sixty years for the FDA to see a connection between their use and deaths among children. That's actually an improvement; it took close to three-thousand years for doctors to see a connection between bloodletting and the subsequent lethal consequences. Unfortunately, the FDA still thinks the problem is parental overdosing not the results of hobbling a useful defense.

Of course, antihistamines, one of our most prevalent allergy, cold, flu and sinus medication families, inhibit the body's production of histamine. There were earlier hints pointing to the dangers of antihistamines, but they were not seen because we were asking the wrong questions. Until around 2001 *The Physicians' Desk Reference* (the big red or blue reference book that tells doctors about the drugs they prescribe) reported on the side effect studies for the drug loratadine (Claritin®), one of the new "non-sedating" antihistamines. Even with less-than-optimal conditions the study of loratadine showed a doubling of both URIs and wheezing during its two-week course. However, this result was considered not statistically significant. If this study had been done in the winter cold season when a fourth or a third of the students are commonly out with colds, and the same doubling held, we would not likely have this drug. An interesting question that no one is going to fund is to see if the flu or now a COVID-19 infection is more serious in people who have taken safe, over-the-counter (OTC) cold pills to deal with the symptoms of their cold.

ASTHMA AND EAR INFECTIONS RISE

In 1992, the National Center for Health Statistics published data showing the increases in ear infections between 1975, when there were ten-million cases, and 1990 when there were twenty-five million.

Ear infections have increased five-percent per year ever since the early 1970s, and so have sinus infections according to ear, nose, and throat doctors. Infectious disease specialists have tried to find reasons for the increases in ear infections and look mostly at the sharing of germs at day care centers. Many specialists seem to be at a loss on how to control the problem. Try as best they can, workers in these centers cannot keep up with the children as they share their toys with all of the bacteria and viruses from their runny noses. Within days a new bacteria generally spreads to every child in a center. Daycare centers are recognized in the health care industry as social cesspools. It makes sense to close them and schools in the face of an epidemic. It's not so easy with nursing homes and workplaces, which are sometimes almost as bad.

The data for asthma also show regular increases, but the underlying reasons are accepted as being more complex. Left out of this complexity, however, is any sense that it may be the fault of the system. A recent observation adding to the complexity is that the asthma increases seen in the west are not seen in eastern bloc countries such as Russia and Albania.

The most complete information on the increases in asthma from the whole country comes from the CDC where they have collected information on asthma prevalence since the 1980s. This data is represented in Figure 3.1.

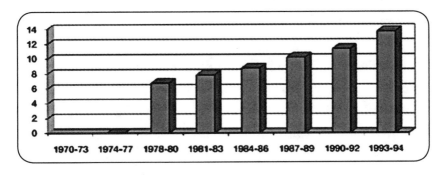

Fig 3.1 *Self-Reported Asthma in Millions*

More telling is data on hospital admissions for asthma collected by researchers at the Medical University of South Carolina in Charleston. They reported hospital admissions for asthma by race going back to 1956, represented in Figure 3.2. The authors of this study, seeing the stable baseline that extended throughout the 1960s, tried to find a reason for the increases that began in the 1970s. They looked at changes in pollution, new industries, and changes in plant pollens; following the pattern of western medicine they looked at all of the things that were outside of the patient—and they could not find anything. They finally looked at the parallel increases in obesity during that time period and concluded there must be a connection. What they failed to see was the correlation with the drugs we now know cause more deaths in children.

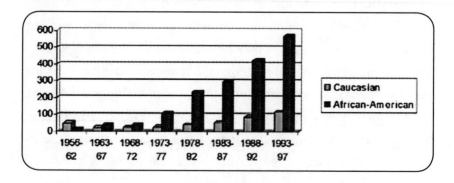

Figure 3.2 *Asthma Discharges from Medical University Hospital in South Carolina*

Cough and cold medicines, the ones withdrawn from use for children in the fall of 2007, are mostly antihistamine and decongestant combinations. They were the miracle drugs of the 1940s. We had learned in the 1930s that histamine was the cause of Johnny's runny nose, and in the 1940s we developed antihistamines that stopped it. It was a wonderful advance because we could now give our children a dose of medicine to get rid of the symptoms and take them to daycare without missing a day of work. But a runny nose, rhinorrhea in medical terms, is there to wash the irritant out of the nose. That's commonsense; our nose doesn't run except when it is irritated. But what happens when we turn off this defense by using cough and cold medicines? Blocking the runny nose with loratadine doubled both the rate of URIs and the incidence of wheezing, and their comparison study with one of the older "sedating" antihistamines showed it to cause even more wheezing. Are the results from the Medical University of South Carolina in Charleston study related to what these drugs do? Many biologists are beginning to see this connection.

The 1970s saw several things happen that greatly enhanced these drugs' use. First of all they had been available by prescription since the 1940s. In 1965, they were deemed safe enough by the FDA to be made available without a prescription. Second, the wide use of television provided an optimal means for the pharmaceutical companies to market them; and third, the advent of Medicaid provided a means to get them into the hands of our poorer populations. I began practicing shortly after all this, but drug representatives still delivered samples of these drugs by the boxful to hand out to those needing them. But these connections are circumstantial; they're not enough for proof. To see how the use of these drugs contributes to upper respiratory problems we have to understand what goes on in the airway when allergens and infectious agents threaten it; and this requires that we see the problem differently.

Christer Svensson, from the Department of Otorhinolaryngology, Head & Neck Surgery, University Hospital, Lund, Sweden, writing in the *American Journal of Rhinology*, saw the role of histamine differently after he looked at what happens in the nose when histamine is released. He saw that it increased both the water in the nose and the mucus, and concluded that its role in the nose is defensive. Histamine, he saw, is the trigger for the back up washing. As with your favorite football team the defense needs to be optimal if you want to win and we believe that seeing our own defenses in this way is better than blocking or hobbling them with drugs when they are bothersome. And while primary defenses are mostly *not* bothersome, back-up defenses generally are. We need to know when our bodies are challenged and, hopefully, when our "service-needed" light comes on we don't just unplug it.

WHY ANTIBIOTICS DON'T WORK WELL ENOUGH ANYMORE

Several years ago my wife and I visited the Great Barrier Reef off the east coast of Australia. We were cautioned, before we dove, against touching any of the reef or animals because they were protected by a biofilm, a viscous material made up of friendly bacteria and their secretions that protected these organisms from viruses, bacteria, and other agents that could infect them. Touching them could potentially remove this biofilm and open them to infection. Of course, anybody who fishes for trout and performs catch and releases knows the same principle applies to their successful survival upon regaining their freedom.

We have the same protective elements working in our bodies; good bacteria live in our noses, gastrointestinal tracts, and our skin—they are everywhere. The good bacteria protect us against many harmful ones by robbing them of places to hold onto as well as food to eat. Some good bacteria even produce antibiotic substances. For example our skin bacteria produce substances to defend against bacteria in our stool, and vaginal bacteria defend against a few of the common pathogens there. As explained earlier the primary defense of the GU-tract is this biofilm community of friendly bacteria. For this reason women who douche regularly open themselves to different bacteria that are not as protective against a variety of infections, from bacterial vaginosis to HIV.

The same holds true for disturbing the friendly bacteria in our noses or GI tracts when we take antibiotics, or, as Dr. Nsouli showed at the end of the last chapter, when we nasal "douche" with a neti pot and vigorously wash out the friendly bacteria. In a way, the protection these friendly bacteria provide even extends outward as our immune systems get used to those bacteria in our environment. Women considering home birthing, for example, are cautioned about the increased possibility of infection if they have not lived in their home for a few months—long enough to get familiar with the bacteria that are present.

When antibiotics were first developed they were very effective. The dose of amoxicillin needed to treat an ear infection was about 250 milligrams (mg) a day for ten days; it's now close to ten times that. Back then we also knew very little about the role bacteria play in the workings of our bodies. Today we know that good bacteria help us live by providing many of the nutrients we need, playing a critical role in many of our primary defenses by providing a shield against bad bacteria, and helping our development, both mental and physical, as we grow.

While our pharmaceutical companies try to make antibiotics that are selective and don't kill the good bacteria, this is largely an effort in futility since there is DNA evidence of hundreds of bacteria in our GI tracts that we have not even identified, let alone added to the list of health friendly species. It is the bacteria in our GI tracts that are mostly those developing resistance. And it's not just our GI-tract bacteria doing this. Animals participate on an even greater scale. In 1954, we made two-million pounds of antibiotics and now we make over fifty million. More than 70 percent of antibiotic production goes to animals where it stimulates the growth of resistance just as it does in humans. Antibiotics are used in animals to prevent epidemics in their unhealthy massive feeding lots, but most use is because antibiotics have been found to promote growth, and when they are sold by the pound that adds a profit incentive—and this part is totally unregulated. Better feed, probiotics, and a cleaner, more natural environment are safer and more effective ways of reducing infections, both in animals and humans.

We need another way to think about this problem. I am by no means saying we should stop using antibiotics; they save lives. But most doctors routinely overprescribe them for many minor or viral infections where they do little good. If we as individuals focus on building our defenses we can get by without taking antibiotics; the friendly bacteria will continue to help us live healthier lives; and if we, as a society, can use antibiotics more responsibly we will have less of a problem with resistant bacteria.

Early on antibiotic resistance was limited to hospitals where antibiotic use was more prevalent and higher dosages were used. But resistant bacteria are now spread around the world, and everyone, even a healthy young person, is open to infection by these super bugs. The way to resolve this major problem is to rely less on our offensive team (antibiotics) and more on strengthening our defenses.

Empowering defenses is not a one-time effort. Creating a habit like regularly washing your hands enhances health. Let me relate a few examples. We have already met JM whose chronic ear infections led to two sets of tubes and surgery to repair a non-closing eardrum. JM was adopted, and he had several siblings who were also adopted. Like JM, they all had medical problems. His mom had a soft spot for kids with problems who would otherwise not have been adopted. Because she was busy with all of her special children she could not spend the time herself to make sure that JM used the spray regularly. When she stopped assisting and monitoring his use, JM's hearing problems returned. Mom had to rededicate herself to JM's regular nasal hygiene routine, and subsequently JM went through the same experience of coughing up of copious amounts of mucus two more times in that year. The spray doesn't cure conditions—it prevents problems. But to do this it has to be used regularly.

Traci's case (the young girl with asthma) demonstrates the same problem. Even though she was able to participate in sports and live free of asthma for several years she stopped using the spray regularly and her asthma did return. It's keeping your nose clean using xylitol that works, and that means regular use. Children are not usually reliable at this, so the guardians or health-care providers have to help them.

Over the years we have found several ways to help in this process:

▶ START EARLY: The spray was designed for a baby and they generally adapt well to its use. Hold the baby upright and spray each nostril, then lay them down and change their diaper so the spray can move to the back of the nose where it is effective.

▶ AVOID DIFFICULTIES WITH COMPLIANCE: Older children become resistant and seek independence. They want to be in control of themselves, which can create problems if you forcefully spray their noses. But this can usually be negotiated. Give them a choice whenever possible, like which side first. When we approach our grandson with the spray he will hold his nose closed and open his mouth. After a spray in his mouth he will open one side of his nose and allow us to spray there. Then we repeat the process for the other side. (The spray is sweet and has a pleasant taste, and if you don't keep it out of their reach many small children will drink it. This doesn't hurt them, but it is not free and it's much more effective if it is passed through the nose than the mouth on the way to the stomach.)

▶ A FAMILY PROTOCOL: By far the best way to promote the use of the spray is for everyone in the household to use it regularly. Children learn by example so if you want them to keep their noses clean you better set a good example.

▶ FREQUENT USE IS ESSENTIAL: Additionally, xylitol chewing gum studies show an optimal benefit of preventing 80 percent of tooth decay when used five times a day; I argue the same for nasal use.

If you or your kids are sick, use the spray often. If you have a chronic condition like allergies, five uses a day is fine, and even less often if you are normally healthy. But regular daily use is essential.

The advice I give to people worried about the flu is appropriate: When you wash your hands wash your nose, and drink enough water. Make sure that happens at least five times a day. I also realize this is ideal and that most people just will not use it that often. People seem to use it when they think about it, i.e. when they start to have a problem. But that may be too late. Take a good look at yourself and your environment. If you are generally healthy and don't have allergies you can likely get away with two to three times a day, but if you have a nasal-related condition or are exposed to a wide variety of infectious agents (like if you are a doctor, teacher, nursing-home, or childcare worker) then you had better find a way to use it more often, and the best way to do that is to associate washing your nose with something you do regularly.

BIOFILM AND INFECTIONS

Both Traci and JM (cases 2 and 15) share another aspect of this story that bears looking at before leaving this subject. They both had episodes where they got rid of a bunch of foreign material in the back of their noses that was associated with their immediate improvement. What's going on here?

I wasn't there, and they didn't bring any of this stuff for me to look at, so this is mostly conjecture on my part, but it makes sense. We have already talked about biofilm and how it protects us and other animals. But there is also a down side. All bacteria can make biofilm, not just the friendly ones. When bad bacteria build biofilm it becomes a safe house for them to hide in. Biofilms are very difficult to remove; it takes a hundred times the normal dose doses of antibiotics to reach bacteria in their safe houses. That amount of antibiotics is enough to kill the person. To add to the problem, typically biofilm infections are cyclical. Chronic otitis is a good example, but certainly not the only one. The fever and other symptoms of infection usually disappear with antibiotics as the bacteria retreat to their safe houses. But the whole thing begins all over as the antibiotic is completed and the environment is safe for the bacteria to begin exploring again.

We know, first of all, how biofilm is formed. When bacteria get into the body the first thing they must do is find a place to hold onto. If they can't hold on they are washed out by the fluids bathing our bodies, and we have no problem. They can multiply if they find a way to hold on and are not recognized early on by our immune systems. As they increase in number, they make a chemical that acts as a signal when it reaches a certain concentration. The process is called quorum sensing and triggers some of the bacteria to start making biofilm—some, but not all. Just as in the case of bacteria mutating to find a means of coping with an antibiotic, for all of them to begin building a biofilm would be suicidal. People studying this process with powerful microscopes describe biofilm in terms reminiscent of a Star Wars city. These bacterial homes are what protect the marine life as well as us when they are made up of helpful bacteria. When they are made up of harmful bacteria they cause long-term problems like chronic infections because the bacteria can stay inside their safe houses where the antibiotics can't reach them.

We were recently visiting our foster son in Sweden, and Jerry began talking with one of his friends, a medical student, about her favorite subject of ear infections. In Sweden, he explained, they find that viruses cause most chronic ear infections so they don't use antibiotics to treat them. She tried to explain the concept of biofilm to him, but it was new and unfamiliar, and he wasn't receptive. I wasn't there to lend her support, but what he was relying on are the studies where they take fluid from the middle ear of children with chronic ear infections and culture it to look for bacteria, and often they don't find any. It is easy to conclude from these studies that bacteria are not there so the infections must be viral, but that conclusion leaves out some significant information.

When fluid is taken from acutely infected middle ears the most common finding is both bacteria and viruses, and this is true for one-time infections or acute flare-ups in those with chronic otitis. And often the bacteria found in the acute flares of chronically infected ears are the same strain, which suggests that these recurrent infections may actually be the same infection. If fluid from these ears is cultured in between acute infections nothing is found, supporting what the Swedish medical student was arguing. But what if the bacteria causing these flares are just hiding out in their biofilm safe houses and are not exposed to the antibiotic used to treat the acute infections? This was a question asked by a group at Pittsburgh who used DNA marking as a means of detecting bacterial biofilm. This test was positive 100 percent of the time when the middle ear fluid from children with chronic ear infections was examined, and 92 percent of the time when they looked at specimens of the middle ear surface membranes. While I was not there and the material they coughed and vomited up was not examined, I believe the cleansing episodes Traci and JM experienced were likely caused by the breaking loose of their biofilm.

OTHER PROBLEMS TOXIC BIOFILMS CREATE

I was thinking about this problem several years ago when I heard Randy Wolcott, one of our local doctors, talk about his work helping wounds to heal. Biofilm, populated with harmful bacteria, is a major problem because it always grows over open wounds and hampers healing. Dr. Wolcott was dealing with wounds of people with insufficient blood supply due to hardening of the arteries or diabetes; if he could not get the wounds to heal the treatment was generally amputation of the limb with the problem.

After his presentation I talked with him about my ideas with xylitol and bacterial adherence, and he began experimenting on his own. The best results on getting these wounds to heal had been in the 65-percent range. Over the subsequent years he found that he could heal 77 percent of these wounds using a dressing containing significant amounts of xylitol and another naturally occurring antibiotic substance called lactoferrin. His nurses, the ones that took care of the wounds, told him that the wounds where the accumulated material at the wound surface would just come off with the dressing always healed. The Center for Biofilm Engineering at the University of Montana participated in this study and their director, Garth James, told me that their experiments showed that xylitol has a broad-spectrum ability to block biofilm formation and adherence. This has since been confirmed by Dr. Wolcott and his group working in Lubbock. Using a wound model with many different types of bacteria, they showed that a 20-percent solution of xylitol stopped all biofilm formation. So now I feel a lot more comfortable thinking that this is what happened with these two children.

A NEED FOR BALANCE

Both good and bad bacteria build biofilm after they first find a way to hold on and are able to multiply. While we need to do something about the bad bacteria and their biofilms, we also desperately need to realize the nature of the symbiotic relationship we have with our friendly bacteria. We could not live without them—not even the ones that cause harm to us. We need to find another way to persuade them not to attack us while we are still alive. We need to find a way to keep our kids out of special education. Avoiding putting tubes in children's ears would certainly save us some serious medical treatment dollars and preventing the infections and the hearing problems that often accompany them would reduce much of our special education needs. In order to do this we need to understand the nature of our nasal defenses and how to support them.

CHAPTER FOUR

Moisturizing with Xylitol

L ike the connection between ear infections and special education, something connects cold weather and illness, but we are not sure what it is exactly. We all recognize that winter season is the time for colds and flu, but hardly anyone asks why. Those that do concentrate again on the bugs. Viruses can survive longer in cold air, which is the proposed reason why flu season doesn't exist in the tropics.

When the colds and flu do come around, everyone seems to have their own favorite treatment designed to thwart the wintertime bugs. The success of these treatments is perceived by a good outcome but could just as well be luck. Few look at how the weather affects our defenses, but my experiences, both in practice and travel, convince me that an underlying reason for the connection between illness and a cold front has to do with humidity and its role in the nasal defenses.

One of those trips was to some small towns in Alaska where we talked with the people who were trying to cope with the ear infections in the native population. This population has the highest incidence of ear infections in the country and quite possibly the whole world.

To review, ear infections are the classic upper respiratory infection for children. Bacteria first come into the nose, and then climb down their eustachian canals into the middle ear where they multiply and cause their problems.

We talked with audiologists and their helpers who went out into the native communities and spoke with the people. They repeatedly heard from the elders in these villages that their people did not have ear infections before they were "civilized." When we asked the doctors about this story they said that the ear infections were there, but they were just not recognized. I am not sure about that. Ear infections are painful and, if not taken care of, only get better when the eardrum ruptures and the puss from the middle ear drains out. That's a pretty easy process to recognize. Furthermore, in a sister city across the Bering Strait in Siberia, the same genetic base that included this disposition for ear infections had neither the benefits of civilization nor the same problem at the time we were there. In all fairness to the doctors, their visits to the frontier "hardship" areas are generally quick, and they have little time to listen to the elders.

"Civilized" meant that they were taken from their ice homes and given prefab houses in which to live. The new furnaces in each home, by heating the air significantly, reduced the relative humidity in their environment.

While this new homes were more comfortable, they significantly altered the environment to which their bodies had adapted. Elders from other native groups, from the aborigines of Australia and New Zealand to the Native Americans of New Mexico, tell the same story: taking people from their native habitat makes them less healthy; and mostly the poor health is centered in the respiratory system. What's going on here?

Besides filtering and cleaning the air that we breathe, the nose also has to warm and humidify it. It normally does this so well that the air entering the lungs is almost always body temperature and 100-percent humid in a variety of environments. In cold environments this is a challenge that requires a great increase in blood circulation to the nose and almost constant flow of small amounts of histamine to help produce fluid. This fluid replenishes the airway-surface liquid layer, which plays an important role in the nose's function. Similar challenges face anyone living outdoors in a temperate environment. Though the challenges exist, people have adapted to them over thousands of years.

The airway surface fluid plays a critical part in helping the cilia and mucus to work best and it interacts with the air we breathe: it is replenished in moist air and reduced in dry air. In the tropics, where the humidity is most often in the healthy 40- to 60-percent range, the nose works better. In the temperate zones, the humidity fluctuates more outside, but, inside, when the central heating/cooling is on, the humidity is generally in the 20- to 30-percent range. This mean that the airway surface fluid has to make up the difference; if the person is not adequately hydrated, the cleaning defenses in the nose become limited.

Most of the fluid needed for this warming and humidification comes from what we drink, but some comes from the environment. Some time ago some people looked at the effect of humidity on our illnesses. This study, together with what we have learned about how our airway defenses work, is why we think humidity is a more defining reason for why we have a flu season.

The chart on the next page (Figure 4.1) shows that while high humidity is associated with more viruses and bacteria it is not associated with more infections; it's only when the air is dry that upper respiratory infections are increased. If there is enough moisture the nose can more easily wash the infecting agents out.

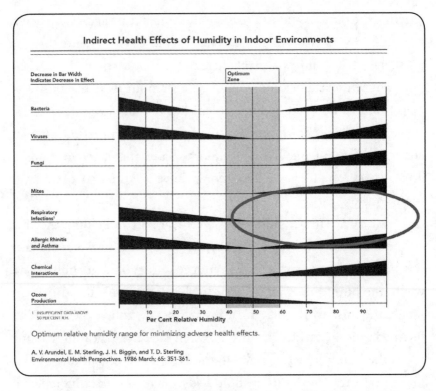

Figure 4.1 *Indirect Health Effects of Humidity in Indoor Environments*

The process for most of moving indoors and into our centrally heated and air-conditioned environments has been slow enough that we did not notice this change in respiratory problems. However, the Alaskan natives did experience problems with the abrupt change in their environment.

Regions in the world greatly affect the humidity in the air. People in the tropics live mostly with the windows open and the humidity is usually in a healthy range. People living in the temperate zones have lower temperatures and must create their own ways to moderate their environment to make it comfortable. Before central heating, they generally lit a fire to warm up. While the heat made the air drier, enough air came in from outside to keep the environment somewhat humid. When central heating emerged, we also diminished drafts in houses, which consequentially lowered the humidity. In a well-insulated home with the central heating on, we have a hard time getting the humidity above 30 percent.

Insulation in homes, isolation from outdoors, and the efficiency of our heating and cooling systems have emerged only within the past fifty years. It takes thousands of years for our bodies to adapt to physical changes in our environments, and we have not had long enough for our noses to adapt to our drier but more comfortable environments.

We need to take other actions to support the defenses we have handicapped in this process. If we don't, we will continue having our cold and flu season, more URIs, and no relief in our battle with allergens and asthma.

Water, after air, is the most critical element for a properly functioning body, and most of us need to make a conscious effort to drink more. It's also the most critical element in the mucociliary elevator, the system of mucus and cilia designed to clean the nose.

CILIA, MUCUS, AND FLUID

If we could look with a microscope inside an ideal nose, we would see all of the pollutants and infecting agents such as bacteria and viruses stuck in mucus that coats and protects our airway. The mucus, which is a tool of our mucosal immune system, would be moving slowly toward the back of the nose. Ideally, it takes about fifteen minutes for the mucus to move from the front of the nose to the back of the throat where we swallow it. Then the acid and digestive enzymes in our stomach recycle all of the proteins in the mucus and destroy the pollutants.

The mucus in our nose is secreted in very concentrated form by special cells scattered among those lining our airway, and it absorbs up to two-hundred times its weight in water, which it gets from the airway surface fluid, to become the sticky, wet substance that captures all of the pollutants. It can hold onto most of the pollutants because of adhesion molecules that cover the mucin chains. These adhesion molecules are a very large variety of sugar complexes that go along with the very large variety of sugar receptors on the surfaces of bacteria—which also helps explain why xylitol works to help. The mucus, with all its pollutants, is swept by microscopic hairs called cilia that grow out of cells in the airway. They normally move back and forth in a waving motion about ten times per second. Between this mucus layer and the ciliated and mucus-secreting cells is the airway surface fluid that has three functions: it provides some space so the cilia can sweep effectively; it acts as a liquid bed for the mucus to float on so it can be easily swept out; and it is the fluid the mucus needs to thin out. The airway surface fluid is also the home of several protein substances, called defensins, which help trap and kill foreign bacteria.

These three elements, the mucus that does the trapping, the cilia that sweep it out, and the airway surface fluid that enables both to work effectively, make up what is called the mucociliary elevator (see Figure 4.2 on the next page)—the primary defense for cleaning the airway. This system cleans practically everywhere in the upper- and lower-respiratory tissues, from the nose to the lungs, and even the eustachian canals. In all areas it moves the mucus to the back of the throat where we swallow it. It works twenty-four hours a day and seven days a week. It is a very effective cleaning mechanism when it is working properly.

Insufficient water results in depleted airway surface fluid, preventing the mucus from becoming wet and sticky. Water is the body's oil; just as oil is a necessary part of all machines, the body needs water. Few of us drink the recommended three to four quarts a day.

When the defenses of the nose are compromised, viruses and bacteria accumulate, take hold, and form colonies that are called biofilms.

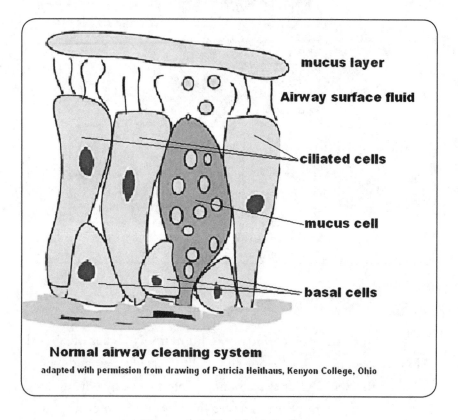

Figure 4.2 *The Nose's Defenses*

These eventually break off and enter the deeper tissues of the lungs, as shown in Figure 4.3 (next page). We are fortunate if we have more than 30-percent humidity in our insulated and centrally heated homes. Adding to the humidity with a humidifier, vaporizer, or even a pot of water on the stove can be helpful. It is also expensive, energy intensive, and, in my own case, has led to many burned-out pots. Using a humidifier requires regular cleaning to prevent molds.

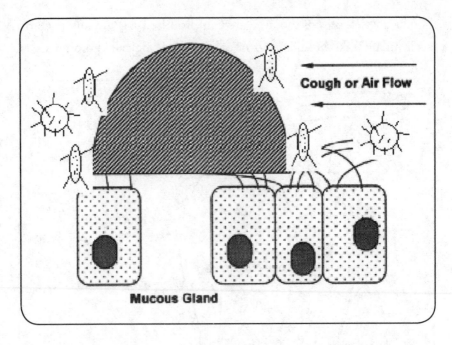

Figure 4.3 *The Nose's Defenses When Impaired*

Moving to the tropics where the humidity is higher offers little help today because we take our air conditioners with us, and cooling the air in this way also dries it. Swamp coolers work by putting water into the air and are healthier in dry environments, but they don't work well in most of the country, or most of the tropics where summer air is both hot and wet.

To moisten dry airways many people use small bottles of saline. These sprays became popular around the same time the use of antihistamines was increasing. Saline sprays do a reasonable job countering the dry nose these drugs cause. They even help reduce the incidence of infections. Researchers at Harvard University found that "heavy polluters," who breathe out large amounts of viruses and bacteria, have, within minutes, less impact by simply inhaling vaporized saline. This happens of course because the mucus is stickier for a few minutes.

If saline is effective at reducing the bacteria we breathe out, one would think that it should also reduce respiratory infections—and it does but not by much. My own experience is characteristic. I began using a nasal saline spray soon after I began dealing with the occupational hazard of respiratory infections in my practice. Saline sprays didn't eliminate the problem, but they did cut it by about a third. Because of this benefit I have recommended the use of these sprays often and aggressively in children with ear infections, but they didn't seem to help at all in these problems. Something else was needed.

Several years ago a group of researchers at Johns Hopkins were looking at the effect of cold air on the nose. Cold air cannot hold as much moisture as warmer air so it tends to dry the airway surface fluid and make what is left more concentrated. In order to mimic this condition they got volunteers to put five milliliters (about a teaspoon) of a concentrated solution of mannitol (a close form of the sugar mannose that is common in the body) into their nose and hold it there for a few seconds before letting it drain back out. When they examined what came out they found that it had more volume. The mannitol had pulled more fluid into the nose. Additionally, there was a small amount of histamine present. When one realizes that histamine is the trigger for the back-up nasal washing and that it is, as Dr. Svensson pointed out, a critical part of the nasal defense, its presence is perfectly understandable. The task of hydrating and warming air requires increased blood flow, which histamine triggers. Consider also that the concentrated mannitol pulls fluid into the nose from the cells in a manner that is functionally identical to histamine.

Osmotic agents such as mannitol are very useful in washing the airway. The fluid they pull into the nose goes into the airway surface fluid where it can be used to adequately hydrate the newly secreted mucus as well as provide a space in which the cilia can more effectively sweep. This shows there is something more effective than just saline.

OSMOSIS WITH XYLITOL

A group at the University of Iowa Carver College of Medicine, with whom I am in correspondence, has researched xylitol's osmotic effect. Shortly after the Finns demonstrated anti-adherence ability, the researchers looked at its use to treat children with cystic fibrosis. They looked a bit further at what xylitol does in the airway and found that it acts locally as an osmotic agent that pulls water into the airway. This is good for most children with cystic fibrosis because their mucus is dry and doesn't work very well. Consequentially, they get upper and lower respiratory infections all of the time, and most of these children die early because of them. These researchers, however, used nebulized xylitol, which is usually inhaled through the mouth and therefore bypasses the nose.

This group looked specifically at the effect of xylitol on the airway surface fluid. They found that more fluid lowers the salt concentration and helps the antibiotic defensins work more effectively. Defensins are small proteins in the airway surface fluid that help rid the airway of infectious agents. Too much salt, however, interferes with their efficacy, which is the case with kids who have cystic fibrosis. Xylitol also provides water for improved thinning of the mucus and more volume so that the cilia can move more effectively.

Osmosis, remembering from high school chemistry, is the movement of water to a more concentrated solution.

The Iowa team also found that the xylitol was not absorbed, which adds to its safety profile. Since xylitol it is not absorbed, it gets moved to the back of the throat and swallowed.

Additionally, when a solution of xylitol was regularly nasally inhaled by a group of volunteers it substantially decreased the number of bacteria in their airway. After four days of regular use, the reduction in bacteria was six-times greater in those sprayed with xylitol than sprayed using only saline. This finding does much to support and explain my own experience on saline not working well.

Finally, the researchers confirmed that xylitol did not aid the growth of a wide variety of harmful bacteria.

Later studies done by this group on the airway surface fluid in the bronchi show that xylitol stays around for about four hours. This supports and explains our finding that frequent use is more helpful.

After all these discoveries, the researchers applied for and were granted a patent for aerosolized xylitol by which it is delivered to the lower airway by breathing with a nebulizer. This route can more easily lead to profitable patenting, because nebulizers are already controlled as medical devices.

But it is not just this osmotic effect that optimizes nasal cleaning with xylitol; another aspect of xylitol is just as important.

XYLITOL AND BACTERIAL ADHERENCE

I already mentioned that I called Dr. Uhari, the lead researcher in the chewing gum/ear infection study, after I found out how putting xylitol in the nose was so much more effective in preventing ear infections than its oral use. Besides encouraging me to reproduce his studies, he told me about a study his group had done that was awaiting publication. This report showed why xylitol was so effective nasally.

This study was done in the laboratory and not in people. Dr. Uhari took cells from the nose and helped them to grow creating an artificial nose. These are the cells that bacteria learn to hold on to when they establish a home in the back of the nose. Then the researchers selected bacteria that cause the most infections. Of these bacteria, they chose strains of bacteria that are the most malicious. Then they took half of each and exposed it to xylitol for a period of time, followed by washing to remove what was not holding on. Then they created four separate groups: one with no xylitol in either cell or bacteria; one with xylitol in both, and; one each with xylitol in either the cell or the bacteria. After some time they counted the number of bacteria holding onto each cell. They found that xylitol has an effect on the adherence of these major nasal pathogens, but mostly on the major pathogen, *Streptococcus pneumoniae*, where the combination of xylitol on both bacteria and cells significantly reduced the ability of these bacteria to hold on, as shown below in Figure 4.4.

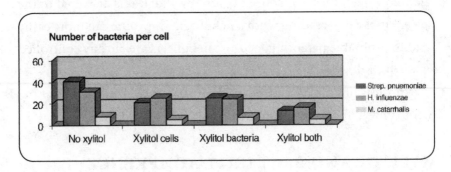

Figure 4.4 *Xylitol's Anti-Adherence Properties*

What bacteria hold on with are numerous molecular-sized hands called lectins that are shaped specifically for their particular receptors. Receptors are what they hold on to. These receptors are almost always specific sugar complexes, like the ones mentioned earlier that are found in nasal mucus. They are also on the surfaces of our cells. Nathan Sharon, one of the earliest researchers to look at this adherence mechanism, said the lectins have a sweet tooth.

HOW SUGARS CAN TREAT INFECTIONS

Dr. Sharon looked at the way *E. coli* adheres in the bladder. These are the bacteria that cause most urinary tract infections (UTIs). He found that they stick to mannose molecules, which are plentiful on the cell surfaces in the genital tract and the bladder. He also suggested that putting mannose in this environment would compete at these binding sites and fill up the bacterial lectins so they could not hold on to the bladder. It's a well-known process called competitive inhibition, and it works. But mannose is one of the more common sugars found in the body and cannot be patented, so again: no patent—no profit; no profit—no research; no research—no drug, and no one knows.

Fortunately there is a sugar that works about a tenth as well as mannose that is available and well-known for this purpose. Grandmother's advice to her daughters to drink cranberry juice to prevent urinary infections most likely works on this basis. There is hardly any mannose in cranberry juice but there is lots of fructose, and fructose has been shown to compete at *E. coli* binding sites, but not as well as the mannose does.

Drinking cranberry juice is not a very effective way to get it into the bladder where it can act directly on these bacteria, but this may not even be necessary. Most UTIs in women begin from bacteria in their own GI tracts. The bacteria get into the bladder because of poor hygiene or can even migrate in bath water. If the GI tract is their reservoir, then addressing the problem there should be just as effective; and research shows that it is. As the person eats the fructose, or drinks the cranberry juice, the infection causing bacteria latch on to this sugar and cannot then hold on in the bowel. They are gradually replaced by strains of bacteria that don't hold on to these sugar complexes and can't cause urinary tract infections.

There is also one study that shows long-term benefits of this concept. Long-term benefits mean that the benefits continue after the treatment ends. They mean that either the bacteria are not there anymore, or they have changed in their nature and do not cause the problem any longer. Taking an appropriate antibiotic for an infection confers a long-term benefit because the infecting bacteria are gone, but it has the downside of stimulating antibiotic resistance and killing off friendly bacteria that decreases their diversity—and our health— as well as the ones causing the infection. There is no downside to using sugars to negotiate with bacteria.

The same group in Finland that did the ear-infection study on xylitol performed another study that showed these long-term benefits in treating urinary infections. They looked at women who had chronic urinary infections that kept coming back despite their regular use of antibiotics. The year long study used a combination of lingonberry and cranberry extracts. Unfortunately, the producer of the extract went out of business halfway through the study. This resulted in an accidental, but very interesting, result. These women were only treated for six months, while they could get the extract, but they were watched for a year—long enough to show that they received a long-term benefit (see Figure 4.5).

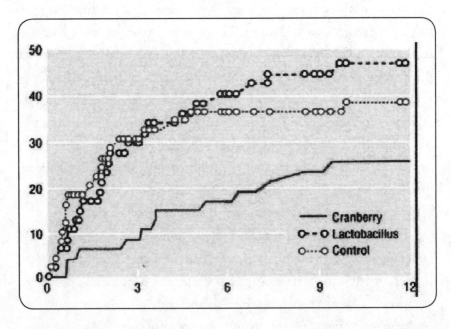

Figure 4.5 *The Lasting Effects of Lignonberry and Cranberry on UTIs*

Many researchers and professionals believe the cranberry juice's mechanism for reducing UTIs is by acidifying the urine, which kills the bacteria. If this were reality then these women should have begun getting infected again after they ran out of the extract.

But they didn't. They received a long-term benefit; the bacteria either shaped up or shipped out.

We will look again at long-term benefits when we talk about xylitol and tooth decay and, again, when we talk about warfare with bacteria. It is an important topic that is not understood in our current model where the focus is on destroying our enemies. It helps us to understand a better way of dealing with our pathogens—and xylitol plays a large part.

Dr. Uhari's study was not the first to show xylitol's ability to block bacterial adherence. Earlier studies by researchers in the Netherlands showed it blocks the adherence of *Clostridium difficile*, bacteria that contaminate poultry, in particular, and often cause food poisoning in the GI tract. Later studies by Japanese researchers showed it blocks the adherence of several strains of staphylococci, even multi-drug-resistant *Staphylococcus aureus*. Add the anti-adherence effect of xylitol to its ability to break up biofilms and you can get a sense of what xylitol can do to help our defenses. It is like soap for the nose—it prevents the bacteria and harmful biofilm from sticking to tissue and brings in more water by its osmotic effects to more effectively wash them all out.

CHAPTER FIVE

Eliminating Allergies and Asthma

I n most areas of the body there are levels of defense, and the nose is no exception. Our primary defenses, like the bacteria, acid, and enzymes in our stomachs and intestines, work without our noticing—until something goes wrong. When our primary GI defenses get overwhelmed, the backstop is gastroenteritis—nausea, vomiting, and diarrhea. Similarly the primary defense in the nose is the combination of the mucus holding on to the pollutants and the cilia sweeping it out, which goes on continuously without our awareness. The backup is more of the same plus the irritation that leads to sneezing and the airway constriction that is asthma, which are bothersome and that our pharmaceutical industry focuses on turning off.

Consider that the most common triggers for asthma are actually allergens that look to the immune system like life-threatening toxins (as in the case of cholera), airborne pollutants, and infectious agents like bacteria or viruses. Margie Profet, an evolutionary biologist who studied at Harvard and the University of California, Berkeley, has shown how allergens share many characteristics with serious toxins and concludes that the response they trigger is a defense with a survival value. Paying attention to these toxins is what has led to one of the more common explanations of allergy yet.

THE HYGIENE HYPOTHESIS

Several years ago researchers looking at allergies in European military recruits found that the problem was significantly less in recruits from rural farms where the barn and animals are adjacent to the house. These and other researchers pursuing this idea concluded that the significant exposure of serious toxins in children kick-started the child's immune system to develop in a healthier way. The idea is known as the hygiene hypothesis, and it is rapidly becoming accepted as a reason for allergies. It explains why we cannot survive well in an extremely sterile environment. The recognition of what is a serious toxin by our immune systems can be especially problematic when we live in a clean environment and have not been exposed to the normal bacteria, pollens, and molds that are more common in less clean households and farming environments. An underdeveloped immune system that has not been exposed to a variety of toxins is more likely to consider allergens or irritants of lesser significance to be real dangers. This association has become apparent in many studies over the last few decades, and, of course, more allergies means more asthma.

If an underdeveloped immune system is overwhelmed by harmless irritants, then the back up is needed.

Part of that is shutting down the airway to protect the more vulnerable lungs from the wrongly identified toxins in the upper airway. And that, I believe, is what happens with asthma. That is why washing the nose is such an effective means of preventing asthma. It addresses the source of the problem.

The chemical that triggers the closing of the airway is histamine—the same histamine that causes the runny nose, itchiness, and sneezing. It's also the same chemical all cold pills (antihistamines) try to block.

Histamine is the trigger for the backup defense—and the defense is both the runny nose and the shutting down of the airway to protect the lungs. Society has turned this reaction into an illness called asthma.

Obviously, no one questions the need for a good doctor during an acute episode. Yet to believe turning that defense off permanently or semi-permanently will cure the patient is also wrong thinking.

There are two ways one can think about these defenses. On the one hand, there are those believing that we were created by God the way we are. On the other hand are those who believe that we are the product of natural selection or evolution. Either way you look at it, these defenses are the best that are available; either God created them or they are expressed in us because of their success. To treat them appropriately we need to honor and support them, even when they are bothersome—and certainly not turn them off.

ONE-AIRWAY HYPOTHESIS

Researchers are looking at the question of how asthma is triggered, but it is slow going. Among some theories is the "one-airway hypothesis," which is based on the well-demonstrated fact that nasal irritants trigger a physiological response that results in bronchospasm, or the constriction of muscles in the bronchioles. People studying asthma have some difficulty with the concept that the major triggers for asthma are in the nose, but this is what my patients tell me. They are not any different from all of the others suffering from asthma. The major triggers are allergies, sinus conditions, and viral upper respiratory infections—all problems that begin in the nose. When the nasal immune system identifies one of these irritants that it cannot wash out, even though it tries (as any person with allergic rhinitis can readily attest), it must focus on limiting the damage by preventing it from getting into the deeper parts of the body. And thus goes the cycle. Reflexes, as pointed out earlier, are always defenses that protect us, and the nasal-bronchial reflex that protects our lungs from perceived pollutants in the upper airway is a defense—asthma is a defense. We have been looking at the wrong aspects of asthma for the last fifty years. That's not very flattering to all of our researchers who are not attracted to this idea. But I can't explain the benefits any other way.

The stand-up comedian Chris Rock is known for a routine where he argues that doctors will never find a cure for AIDS as long as they make money off of treating it. A profit shifts the focus from prevention to making the symptoms livable. In some respects it's the same with asthma. The focus is on making the symptoms livable so few see the role of a clean nose in preventing the problem.

WASH YOUR NOSE

I attended a conference entitled "Rethinking the Pathogenesis of Asthma" some years ago in Santa Fe, New Mexico, where I presented some of these ideas. One of the speakers was Dr. Stephen Holgate, the British Medical Research Council Clinical Professor of Immunopharmacology and Honorary Consultant Physician within Medicine at the University of Southampton and recognized authority on the origins of asthma. He pointed out three things in his presentation: we have gone thirty years with no new treatment for asthma; asthma is caused by injury to the airway; and what we need is a way to protect the airway from this injury. I told him the best way to protect the airway is to wash your your nose.

But this concept requires that we think differently about asthma and that is hard to get across, especially to the professionals who make their living treating this disease.

The hygiene hypothesis is increasingly accepted, though, because the evidence is so pervasive, but there is much foot dragging. Asthma is a condition that is hard to explain in the traditional view of modern allopathic medicine, where one deals only with airway inflammation and constriction, without asking why. One can address both of these elements with drugs like steroids that block the inflammation and bronchodilators to open the airway. Both allow patients to live with the illness and continue to bring profit to the industry. I have seen that orientation in both health professionals (who decline to look at what a clean nose would do to conditions like asthma) and by medical researchers (who would see their pharmaceutical research money disappear). The point here is that regularly washing the nose reduces exposure to our environmental pollutants and allows the body to both learn about and better deal with these threats, both from allergens and infectious agents, without the challenge being too great.

When children are exposed to toxins in this manner, their immune systems have little trouble recognizing the bad guys; their immune systems become educated, and they learn that ragweed or cedar are not really as bad as the other toxins. This is also the goal of immunotherapy in allopathic medicine and homeopathy where a small amount of poison is introduced into the body to educate the cells in a more gentle fashion. In the future we may possibly have easy and safe ways to expose our children to these toxins that will help avoid asthma and allergy problems with great effectiveness. In the meantime we need to honor what our immune system is trying to do.

A COUNTRY DOCTOR'S POINT OF VIEW

After the success we saw with Traci and her asthma, I began using the spray more often with asthma patients. An early opportunity came when an eleven-year old boy, with no prior history of asthma, came to my office wheezing with a peak flow of 150, which is not very good. To review, peak flow measures how much air a person can force out, giving a rough idea of the openness of the airway. His airflow improved with an albuterol-breathing treatment, so I gave him a prescription for an inhaler and a bottle of the nasal spray. I told him to clean his nose regularly for a few days. He did not get the albuterol inhaler, but he took the spray to the school nurse and every class break he would spray his nose. His peak flow over the next three days went from 150 to 250, to 350, and to 450, which was normal for his size. You can get the spray that I developed, by the way, from any drug store in America. I've seen its popularity grow because just as it worked in this case it works over and over with other individuals. It is a way, I guess, of my continuing to help my patients. Only now I count patients on just about every continent.

OTHER PROBLEMS THAT HOBBLE BODILY DEFENSES

As discussed before, there are also several factors we have already mentioned that hurt the body's defensive efforts through the mucus and cilia. Smoking impairs the cilia so they don't work properly. It also loads the airway with lots of toxic chemicals. The cilia become disorganized and don't beat effectively, and the airway soon shows indication of irritation and inflammation, For children this is even worse. We don't know which of these factors, the smoke or the toxins, is so damaging to the airway of smaller children, but the message is clear that we should not smoke around them.

Even clearer is the reason for the effect of dryness on your nasal defenses. Figure 5.1 is a representation of this cleaning process when it is handicapped by dryness and when it is at its most efficient and optimal performance level. When the mucus is dry it does not hold on to the bacteria or other pollutants effectively nor is it able to be moved out as easily. The cilia are disorganized, and the airway surface fluid is compromised and deficient. This nose is comparable to one coping with cystic fibrosis.

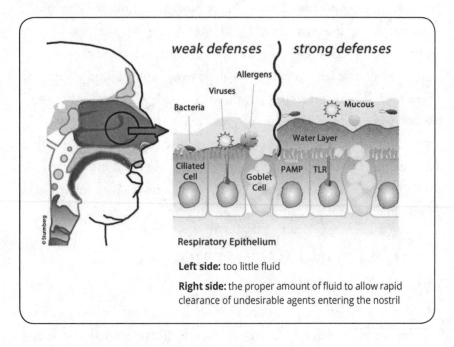

Figure 5.1 *The Cleaning Process*

Your nose's goblet cells secrete mucus in order to protect the mucous membranes. Goblet cells accomplish this by secreting mucins, large glycoproteins formed mostly by carbohydrates. Mucus secreted in the nose rapidly absorbs water to increase its volume by several hundred times, and again, the wetter it is the better it works. It gets this water from the airway surface fluid and if the person is at all dehydrated and the air is dry, a common combination during cold season, the cleaning mechanism is compromised. This underscores the importance of drinking enough water as well as trying to maintain a healthy humidity in the environment for the proper working of this cleaning action.

SCRUBBING-HISTAMINE RESPONSE

Just as some spills on the kitchen floor require more than a broom, there are times when the mucociliary clearance is not up to the job of cleaning the nose. When pollutant sensing cells in the nose are triggered by foreign debris, toxins, or infecting agents they trigger the backup cleaning by releasing histamine. In the 1940s, histamine was labeled a bad molecule. It triggers inflammation. Inflammation is bad. Therefore, histamine was the enemy. Most of our health care industry continues to think this way, but this is naively misleading and circumstantial, and some doctors and scientists are coming around. Christer Svensson, the researcher from Sweden, used his electron microscope to look for any harmful effects in nasal tissue after a histamine challenge and was unable to find any damaging consequences. Dr. Svensson concluded that histamine and the washing it triggers is actually a defense.

According to the American Academy of Allergy, Asthma, and Immunology, histamine does four things in the nose: first, it opens small blood vessels under the cells lining the nasal cavity so they leak; second, it increases the mucus; third, it's an irritant; and finally fourth, it closes the airway.

- ▶ Opening the blood vessels does several things:
  - ○ It provides the water for the washing. The fluid trickles up around the cells, bathing them in the process.
  - ○ It replenishes and increases the airway surface fluid with its defensins.
  - ○ It optimizes the water available for the mucus to be wet, sticky, and moveable, and thus helps it all get cleaned out faster and easier.

- ▶ Increasing the mucus is like adding a vacuum cleaner to the process. More mucus picks up more garbage.

► The local irritation increases the sneezing and, as any mother can readily attest, the socially unacceptable display of mucus coming from the nose is all too often brought on by a sneeze. But would you rather have the pollutants and the mucus holding them in your child's nose or out? This cleaning is a defense and the pollutants it is attempting to remove do cause problems in our bodies.

► The fourth effect of histamine is closing down the airway to protect the more vulnerable lungs.

Cough and cold pills shut down this backup. These pills are made up of decongestants, which close down the opening of the blood vessels and turn off the water. They also have antihistamines, which block the effects of histamine and turn off the whole process. When one goes to the doctor with severe symptoms they are commonly given a shot or a prescription for steroids, which turns off the immune system so it doesn't care if the nose is polluted. Honoring and supporting these defenses is a much better choice than using what is available from the wonders of modern medicine.

Our immune system is strongest in these openings to the body; it is there to recognize, identify, and build defenses against invaders. At the same time it operates throughout our body seeking out abnormal cells like those that turn into cancer. It needs to be optimal, and we should think twice before taking drugs that handicap it or turn it off.

CHAPTER SIX

Taming the Sinus's Wild Beasts

One way to look at xylitol is as the horse whisperer of the bacterial and viral world. Xylitol tames the wild beasts feeding in your nose. This is important. Because our end goal should be to domesticate our bacterial and viral enemies, not vanquish them; we never will, anyway. The war against bacteria and viruses is one we simply won't win. We must learn to live with them. Yet, for allopathic medicine, this is a difficult concept to grasp and implement in one's practice. I was different that way with my patients. I didn't try to bomb their nasal enemies into submission with my vast arsenal of antibiotics. Instead, I taught my patients to tame their enemies.

Warfare has always been a part of our lives in America. We were born of a Revolutionary War, preserved as one nation by a Civil War, and made safe by a series of wars against our foreign enemies. Our bodies are also periodically involved in warfare. Bacteria and viruses regularly invade our bodies and could cause us to be seriously ill were it not for our immune system that deals with most of these agents before they harm us. When we do get signs of an infection, we generally rely on antibiotics to help destroy the invading agents.

Our economy flourishes during wartime. National debt goes up to support the war economy, whether the war is cold or hot. In much the same way the pharmaceutical and health care industries benefit from our warfare with bacteria. But endless warfare is costly and many empires, like the ancient Greeks and Romans, collapsed in large part because of them. There is also a real link in humans between our illnesses and poverty.

Technology has played a large part in who wins our wars. Rifles won out over the bow and arrow, guided missiles over artillery; even the stirrup played a role by giving the mounted warrior more stability. The arms race is the attempt to maintain a position of strength with our enemy. But even when one side is clearly dominant there is always a way to fight back. One-sided, technical superiority breeds unconventional warfare as we have seen with guerrilla uprising we can't seem to quell and terrorism.

Our arms race with bacteria occurs when we use antibiotics to kill the infecting agent and the agent develops ways to get around them. This resistance prompts us to develop the next generation of more potent antibiotics, and the cycle continues. As discussed earlier the race is even manifest in our immunizations; our immunization for pneumonia helps our immune systems recognize and kill the stronger strains of *Streptococcus pneumoniae*. But it is becoming less effective since it just opens the doors for other strains. A similar problem is present with our immunization to whooping cough where bacteria are showing resistance and infections increase. On the other hand our immunizations for tetanus and diphtheria have been around for decades and are still as effective as they were when first developed; and there is no sign of resistant bacteria. The difference between these two types of immunization is that the long-lasting group addresses not the bacteria but the toxins they produce, and the problematic immunizations target the bacteria themselves.

SENSIBLE AND COST EFFECTIVE, BUT NOT GLAMOROUS

Bacteria, like all living agents, sense and adapt to their environments. In fact they are experts in this field. When challenged with antibiotics, or in any other way, bacteria increase their rate of mutation to find a way to cope with the threat. When they are not directly challenged, the bacteria sense no need to adapt. This is the message of Paul Ewald, the evolutionary biologist who says, in *The Evolution of Infectious Disease*, we can "domesticate [bacteria] so that they can live with us in a less damaging way than they have throughout our history."

We can do this, he argues, by shifting how we cope with them. Attacking them leads to resistance, as we have seen. If, instead of attacking them, we address the areas that make it easy for them to get from one person to another, they tend to adapt in friendlier ways.

We did this with cholera by public health measures that cleaned our public water supplies, and we are doing the same for HIV with condoms and needle exchanges. In the case of cholera, cleaning of the water actually changes the agents to types that are less harmful. Dr. Ewald claims the same trend is present with HIV/AIDS in Uganda and Japan where monogamy and condoms are openly and widely promoted. This is the kind of change that leads to the long-term benefits discussed earlier when bacteria change their nature. Epidemic cholera killed millions, but the cholera that has followed cleaning up water supplies is the El Tor strain where the mortality rate is almost negligible.

Anything we can do to create pressure on an infecting agent without it being a threat is a step in the right direction. Isolation does this for all infectious diseases. Window screens do this for diseases carried by insects. Condoms do this for sexually transmitted infections. Washing hands and noses does this for most other socially communicable diseases. We need to promote all of these measures; they are ways we can negotiate in a war we cannot win.

This is even more important because our infectious agents appear to be expanding their range of abilities by fighting back in different ways. When he was the head of the CDC, Dr. David Satcher pointed out that in a twenty-one-year period in the midst of this war, over twenty previously unknown agents or infectious diseases were discovered. Some of these guerrilla fighters are the bacteria that cause ulcers and the virus that causes AIDS, which remain camouflaged while they infect us. One is even a suicide bomber—the Ebola virus kills the host so rapidly that the virus doesn't have time to spread to another person. Now, of course, we must cope with COVID-19. Once again, our defense-based medicine will quell the flames as quickly as possible, in the upper respiratory tract, before they can spread into a brush fire in the lungs.

We have turned bacteria into enemies against whom we must wage all out bomb warfare—bombs being antibiotics. We want them eradicated, so we sell antibacterial soap, and we bleach our countertops to kill germs that are there. The problem is, bacteria are everywhere. Ten percent of our own dry body weight is those bacteria that live with us. At least 50 percent of our DNA is straight from bacteria. Some estimate there are ten times more bacteria in our bodies than the larger cells of which we are made. They are not necessarily evil.

Bacteria are totally responsible for creating the balance that allowed life on this world, and they are primarily responsible for the recycling of materials that maintains that balance. They play a vital role in our defenses by providing barriers and helping in our digestion and making vitamins. Nor are they ignorant. By releasing chemicals that lead to quorum sensing, bacteria are able to communicate with each other and act like a much larger organism. When left alone they make biofilm that is often as elaborate on a bacterial scale as the skyscrapers of New York. They also help each other by sharing genetic information, not only among their own type, but with any bacteria they come in contact with. This cooperation is one reason we are always playing catch-up in the arms race against them.

Nations sometimes fight preventive wars. When under pressure we always go back to our first principles.

But as the German philosopher Georg Wilhelm Friedrich Hegel pointed out in his historical writings, "Institutions are destroyed, in the end, by an excess of their first principles." Sometimes we fight preventive wars with bacteria by taking antibiotics when we are at risk of being infected. Much of our antibiotics are used in the livestock industry for this reason, but also because antibiotics promote growth. This use is largely unregulated. We are finding, however, that the benefit of reduced infections in humans and animals is not worth the cost of the bacterial resistance that comes from the increased exposure to the antibiotic. Nor are they ignorant; even without brains natural selection has taught them to cooperate. The most effective way to stop antibiotic resistance is to reduce our reliance on and use of antibiotics. Fighting unwinnable wars is not a good option on any scale.

We are in an even more helpless position in using "bombs" to fight viruses. Dr. Ewald argues for using actions that block transmission of germs, including viruses such as COVID-19. We argue that using xylitol applies essentially the same pressures, but takes it to the second step. The agent's first step is getting to a new host—the one Ewald addresses. The second is finding a place to hold on in the new host. If the attachment to the new host is foiled then the same pressures are applied that push the bacteria to a more friendly adaptation.

SIMPLE, REASONABLE, AND NOT EVEN TRIED

Dr. Sharon, the biochemist who looked at how bacteria attach to sugar complexes, argued for over twenty years that sugars could be effectively used to prevent infectious disease. Bacteria attach to specific sugar complexes on the cell surfaces in our bodies, and if they can't attach to these sugars they are washed out and don't cause infection. Feeding bacteria with the proper sugars, like those in our nasal mucus, fills up their hungry hands, leaving them with no means of attaching to us. It decreases their adherence to the cells in our bodies. Regular use of such sugars also isolates the infectious agents, and creates a situation much like the *E. coli* and urinary infections talked about previously. Putting sugars, like xylitol and the sugar from cranberries, into the appropriate bacterial environment doesn't kill or threaten bacteria. It just fills up their hungry hands and gives them something to hold on to besides us. Sharon thinks that these sugars may interrupt a part of the bacterial communication system. With an environment filled with the right sugars, what they see is essentially a "shape up or ship out" message, in line with Ewald's observations. This is exactly what we observe when xylitol is present in the nose (and in the mouth). Either the bacteria adapt to a less harmful strain or they are washed out.

This message—to shape up or ship out—is best delivered regularly. So the sugars have to be used regularly even when there is no sign of infection. Women drank cranberry extract every day for six months, but they had protection from urinary infections for a year. To put it in another way, our ancestors, who first fed the wolf cooked meat, had to feed it regularly for a long time before the beast became humankind's best friend. Maybe we can do the same with bacteria. Dr. Ewald thinks it's possible and using the right sugars is a vital part to the process.

Ever since Pasteur discovered bacteria and came up with the germ theory, we have been at war with these microbes. Early on in this war we thought the enemy was only an aggressor that was trying to kill us. It wasn't until relatively recently that we realized how really dependent we are on the bacteria living in us and around us. They are a significant part of the primary defenses in all of those vulnerable open areas of our bodies where their friendly biofilm protects us from countless pathogens. We do know now that killing off all of the bad bacteria is neither practical nor possible. We need these other options. Xylitol for washing your nose is one of the smartest options. Who would have thought that we would be making docile pets of these once predaceous bacterial strains?

Xylitol is like soap for the nose, and a soap that can be used regularly and easily. The frequent use of soap and water on the hands is accepted as the easiest and best way to stop the spread of communicable diseases.

Washing your nose often with a spray containing an adequate amount of xylitol is even easier, better, and more effective. The bacteria and viruses don't get into our bodies through our hands but we introduce them ourselves when we rub our eyes or nose. Of course, we should wash our hands, but it also makes sense to wash the nose.

Sinusitis is one of the most prevalent chronic illnesses in the United States, consistently reported by 13- to 14-percent of adults annually for the last 20 years. More than 250,000 sinus operations are performed annually, making it one of the most frequent surgical procedures after septoplasty (260,000).

In an article in the March 2019 issue of *Otolaryngology—Head and Neck Surgery*, doctors describe the effect of xylitol nasal irrigation in a large sample of patients who had nasal surgery. The study included 100 patients with sinonasal disease who underwent endoscopic sinus surgery (ESS) septoplasty or both concurrently.

Nasal symptoms were evaluated with the NOSE (Nasal Obstruction Symptoms Evaluation) and SNOT-20 (Sino-Nasal

Outcome Test-20). In the ESS group, the general nasal symptom score "showed significantly greater improvement in the xylitol group versus the saline group."

Symptom scores for sneezing, headache and facial pain "were also more improved in the xylitol group."

Nasal stuffiness "showed a significantly greater improvement in the xylitol group when compared with the saline irrigation group."

Among patients with allergic sensitization, rhinorrhea symptoms improved significantly more in the xylitol group than in the saline group.

The preference survey showed that more than half of the patients in each surgical group preferred xylitol irrigation.

The article concluded, "We found that xylitol nasal irrigation was useful in postoperative ESS and septoplasty care. For patients with allergic sensitization, rhinorrhea showed greater improvement in the xylitol group than in the saline group.

In another study from the Department of Otolaryngology— Head and Neck Surgery, Stanford Hospital and Clinics, Stanford, California, to determine the tolerability of xylitol mixed with water as a nasal irrigant and to evaluate whether xylitol nasal irrigation results in symptomatic improvement of subjects with chronic rhinosinusitis, researchers enlisted 20 participants in a prospective, randomized, double-blinded, controlled crossover pilot study.

They were instructed to perform 10-day courses of daily xylitol and saline irrigation in a randomized fashion with a three-day washout irrigation rest period at the start of each treatment arm.

There was a significant reduction in symptom scores during the xylitol phase of irrigation (mean drop of 2.43 points) as compared to the saline phase (mean increase of 3.93 points), indicating improved sinonasal symptoms.

No patient stopped performing the irrigations owing to intolerance of the xylitol, although its sweet taste was not preferred by three subjects (21 percent). One patient reported transient stinging with xylitol. Lead author Joshua D. Weissman M.D., concluded "Xylitol in water is a well-tolerated agent for sinonasal irrigation. In the short term, xylitol irrigations result in greater improvement of symptoms of chronic rhinosinusitis as compared to saline irrigation." Using xylitol for nasal irrigation, however, does not avoid the problems associated with the washing out of the friendly biofilm seen by Dr. Nsouli. We feel that tweaking our bacterial environment with xylitol is far better than trying to wash it out completely.

All of this bears out that regular washing of your nose with a xylitol-based spray solution will not only tame the wild beasts of your nasal passages but end your sinusitis problems too.

CHAPTER SEVEN

The COVID-19 Pandemic, Reframed

I f you have read the earlier chapters you would have read about ORT and how it impacted my early practice. As I mentioned, ORT was used to replace the fluids lost in cholera epidemics and has saved millions of lives over the years—more lives in ten years than penicillin in forty. That should make it a drug, but it isn't. It's made of sugar, salt, and water in the right proportions, which triggers a system in the stomach that pumps water into the body. It saves lives because it optimizes our GI's backup-washing defenses by simply keeping the body's fluid tank full. You can mix it up at home by mixing ¼ teaspoon of salt, 3 tablespoons of sugar, and 1 quart of water (see Resources for more details). If you are dealing with a GI problem start with this and it won't last as long, and you won't have problems with dehydration—which is what kills people with cholera.

The benefits of ORT were researched in the 1950s and 1960s. It was used in studies in the 1970s. The World Health Organization recommended its use in 1978, but without drug status widespread acceptance and implementation was sporadic. Then there was a critical need with a new 1980 cholera epidemic in Bangladesh. BRAC is an international development group based in Bangladesh with the largest number of employees of any non-governmental organization. Among its 90,000 employees, some 70 percent are women. BRAC sent women into all affected communities with a simple, life-saving message for the people: mix a pinch of salt and fistful of sugar in a glass of water, and drink more than you lose. They did this for the whole decade. It was not a randomized double-blind placebo-controlled trial, but it worked—it saved countless lives. And the important lesson is that it worked because it optimized a defense.

This is not an isolated case: a CDC press report dated March 12, 2012 reported that from 1999 to 2007 the mortality rate from GI illnesses in the U.S. grew from 7,000 to more than 17,000 annually. This increase took place in the US alone. The rest of the world knows about and uses ORT for these illnesses and has seen declines in GI mortality. In his history of ORT, published in *Medical History* in 1994, Josh Ruxin clearly points to our profit oriented health-care system as the primary blockade to its use here—when profits and lives are in the balance here in the U.S. profits seems to win.

That lesson is just as important, if not more-so, for our respiratory defenses in a time of the coronavirus. Used appropriately, ORT could save the citizens of the United States thousands of lives and billions of dollars annually. The more prevalent reliance on xylitol as medicine during a time of coronavirus would also save countless lives and offer similar savings when it comes to respiratory health among our citizens. I know that I am but a country doctor and my words are far too modest to excite the political bigwigs in Washington, D.C. and at the CDC in Atlanta. But what I am telling you, especially if you are one of the essential working people, first responders or medical professionals who must grapple daily with the prospect of infection, will help to protect you at your most vulnerable moments in time.

This is possible because xylitol in a nasal spray optimizes this defense in three ways. First of all the water that it pulls into the airway gives the cilia adequate space in which to sweep out viruses and the bacteria on which they so often hitch rides. Second, the water is also absorbed by the concentrated mucus to become the stuff that works. And third, because it is a flexible look-alike to many of the sugars on our cells that the microbes hold on to in order to infect us, it tricks them into holding onto the xylitol rather than the sugars it is looking for on our cells. This is the same thing that the vast number of sugar complexes on our nasal mucins do, and xylitol adds significantly to the process. All of this has to do with how xylitol helps our defenses. We suspect that the aid it supplies to keep our noses hydrated extends to the coronavirus as well.

SO DOES XYLITOL WORK THIS WAY WITH THE VIRUS OR NOT?

That question is being looked at with both xylitol alone and as a synergist when used with another drug. This part of the story is most interesting, and we've learned much more about xylitol during the course of our most recent studies.

When I first began researching xylitol, there was very little experimental, much less clinical, data about its impact on viruses. I still think we have too little experimental and clinical evidence. But a number of experimental studies have shown us that xylitol is a valuable tool not only for influenza but the coronavirus that emerged in late 2019 in Wuhan, China, and is called COVID-19 or SARSCoV-2.

My initial belief in xylitol's usefulness was primarily from an understanding of how viruses enter the body and methods by which the sugar bolsters our mucosal-immune defenses in the nose.

WE ARE ALL VIRAL TAXICABS

One way viruses enter the body is via bacteria. A few years ago I read a book by Lewis Thomas, a physician who thought out of the box enough to turn evolution on its head. He suggested that higher organisms, including humans, may just be technological developments of bacteria to enable them to get around better—bacteria may be taxicabs for viruses, but we may be taxicabs for the bacteria.

Airborne viruses enter cells lining the respiratory tract. Some viruses, like polio and the chicken pox, pick on nerve cells. Others pick on different organs like the liver or brain. All of them, along with all other infecting organisms, appear to follow Paul Ewald's concept of evolving toward living with the host in a peaceful symbiotic relationship if they are sufficiently isolated or, to follow our analogy, if we don't let the taxis stop and unload. He points out that even the virulent strains of HIV Japanese men pick up in Indonesia are tamed when they go back to Japan where condom use is much more prevalent and accepted. Bacteria often enter the body through the nose. But they also often carry viruses with them. They are the taxicab on which viruses ride.

Pollution also matters. Practicing medicine in a region with polluted air from seasonal cotton harvesting and ginning, I have seen firsthand in patients that pollutants are virtual taxicabs for viruses. Besides allergies and asthma, incidence of flu among my patients was always highest when the air pollution was its worst.

Viruses hitch a ride on pollutants to invade our bodies. A study from the Società Italiana di Medicina Ambientale (SIMA) and University of Bologna reported that the spread of the contagious virus in Northern Italy is likely to be linked to air pollution. According to the recent SIMA analysis of COVID-19 diffusion in Italy, the atmospheric particulate matter (PM) exercises a *carrier* (or *boost*) action along with the virus. The assumption that air pollution conditions facilitate the spread of the virus was also previously shown during the SARS outbreak in mainland China in November 2002 when a study analyzed the correlation between PM and the rate of fatalities across five regions. In the US, small increases in long-term exposure to PM led to a large increase in the COVID-19 death rate, say Harvard researchers Xiao Wu and Rachel C. Nethery of the T.H. Chan School of Public Health. "Our results underscore the importance of continuing to enforce existing air pollution regulations to protect human health both during and after the COVID-19 crisis."

Nasal xylitol compensates for much of this pollution by augmenting your body's innate and most primary mucosal defenses in the nose, including drawing in moisture and supporting the cilia in sweeping away the pollutants. It would be better, obviously, for society to deal with pollution at its source. But using xylitol certainly helps.

We also now have experimental research that shows xylitol helps with viruses by not letting them get out of the taxicabs. Even if bacteria sneak into your body, they cannot stick around. I mean literally "stick" around. Microbial adhesion is the first step for colonization or infection. Xylitol makes the terrain of your body way too slippery for disease-causing viruses, bacteria, and fungi to stick around and grow.

No matter whether we're looking at bacteria, fungi, or viruses, these invasive organisms need to be able to adhere to the body's terrain, that is, your tissues, in order to populate and form larger colonies called biofilms.

Researchers have discovered that xylitol can prevent the ability of some tough microbial hombres like Influenza A that cause flu and other respiratory diseases to adhere to the body's tissues. In an experimental study published in the May 1998 issue of the *Journal of Antimicrobial Chemotherapy*, xylitol "reduced the adherence significantly" of *Haemophilus influenzae* and *Moraxella catarrhalis*, which cause diseases of the respiratory system, middle ear, eye, central nervous system, and joints. Proximity is important; the study showed xylitol is particularly effective when both tissues and bacteria came into contact with the sugar. Microbial adhesion is the first step. But if the microbe is holding onto xylitol, it can't hold on to you.

Looking at the effect of xylitol on viruses, a study from *PLoS One* shows that, combined with red ginseng (RG), xylitol offers significant firepower against flu symptoms. Scientists found a "protective effect of dietary xylitol on influenza A infection [(H1N1)]." This H1N1 strain is the one that goes directly to the lungs, but it gets there via the nose, and I wonder if nasal administration would not be more effective.

Mortality in mice infected with influenza A virus could not be influenced by prophylactic oral application of xylitol or RG when used alone. However, combining the two remarkably reduced mortality. Survival against H1NI was "markedly enhanced when xylitol was administered along with RGs, pointing to a synergistic effect. The effect of xylitol plus RG fractions increased with increasing dose of xylitol. Moreover, dietary xylitol along with the RG water soluble fraction significantly reduced lung virus titers after infection. Therefore, we suggest that dietary xylitol is effective in ameliorating influenza-induced symptoms when it is administered with RG fractions, and this protective effect of xylitol should be considered in relation to other diseases."

Human respiratory syncytial virus (hRSV) is the most common cause of bronchiolitis and pneumonia in infants. Nine percent of infant deaths are caused by bronchiolitis and pneumonia. In fact, hRSV is the most common cause of bronchiolitis, a frequently occurring lung infection, and pneumonia in infants.

The effect of dietary xylitol on hRSV infection was investigated experimentally with a 14-day viral challenge. "Significantly larger reductions" in the virus were found in the xylitol group. "These results indicate that dietary xylitol can ameliorate hRSV infections and reduce inflammation-associated immune responses to hRSV infection."

The lack of proper prophylactics and therapeutics for controlling hRSV infection has been of great concern worldwide. Once again, using a xylitol nasal spray would optimize the baby's nasal defenses and be very protective. In my practice, I found that the babies I treated with this problem recovered rapidly when parents used this spray at every diaper change, but I don't know whether that improvement was due to an adverse effect on the virus or a helpful defense effect.

THE SOLUTION FOR COVID-19 IS IN YOUR MEDICINE CABINET

One of the most gratifying aspects of my research into xylitol has been to become part of a growing network of researchers and clinicians from different fields throughout the world who share a similar passion for this unique sugar. We meet at conferences (and hopefully will continue to do so after the current coronavirus pandemic) as well as work together through email, teleconferences, and publications. Through this network, I've worked with doctors in Asia, Europe, South America, Australia, and, of course, North America, Latin America, and the Caribbean.

One of the newer applications for xylitol that some of these doctors have been pushing is combining it with an antihistamine so that some drug claims could be made for the non-drug medication. I was the resistant purist—our use of antihistamines is the underlying problem behind our increases in upper respiratory problems and I wanted nothing to do with them—that is, until the company was approached by one wanting to combine an old antihistamine, chlorpheniramine maleate (CPM), with our xylitol nasal spray. This particular antihistamine was active against Influenza, both A and B and it could work in the nose at far less dosage than in a capsule.

This came to our attention because a Miami pulmonologist, Dr. Gustavo Ferrer, was familiar with the research behind this use of CPM. He contacted Xlear because he needed the xylitol.

The story of CPM and the flu dates from Chinese researchers in 2018 who were looking for ways to deal with the flu and published their research in a peer-reviewed article in *Frontiers in Microbiology*. They found CPM was effective at stopping a variety of flu viruses from entering the vulnerable host cells in our noses. Total protection was given to the mice in their study when the drug was injected prior to infection, and they concluded CPM is a "potent" antiviral. After screening an FDA-approved drug library containing 1,280 compounds, including COVID-19 treatment candidates favipiravir and oseltamivir, for effects against viruses, the article's authors said CPM was far more distinguished than the others and shown to have "potent antiviral activity against a broad spectrum of influenza viruses."

But the flu, while still important for the problems and deaths it causes, was eclipsed by the SARS-CoV-2 that causes our current pandemic, so the company contracted with the Antiviral Research Lab at Utah State University to see if the nasal spray would benefit people with COVID-19.

The problem was the spray they tested had many added natural substances so when the results came back that it killed 75% of the SARS-CoV-2 virus in 30 minutes we were excited, but we needed to know which element was responsible. More testing revealed the active substance to be grapefruit seed extract (GSE), a preservative used to extend the shelf life of the spray and keep the spray free of molds and other substances.

The lab results are in the form of decreases in titer comparing the test substance to both a control and a known killer, like alcohol. The titer is measured in logarithmic terms: the log of the control was 3; the log of both the test substance and the alcohol was less than 0.67—the lab's lower limit of detection. A titer of 3 is 10 to the third power or 1000. In this part of the study, the virus was reduced by more than 99 percent, and it was done in 15 minutes, not 30.

GSE has a very mixed record: the pharmaceutical industry says there is nothing to it—that whatever efficacy it has is due to contaminants (see the write up in Wikipedia); the alternative medical industry says the opposite. Xlear, the company making the spray, reports regularly testing their GSE for contaminants, which have not been found. It's hard to argue with the lab results and their confirmation by an independent lab in Geneva, so we side with the alternatives here as elsewhere. A good reason why is seen in how the mainstream treats the current virus.

Both corona viruses and most influenza viruses enter our bodies via the airway and attach first in the nose. H1N1 flu goes to the lungs. Infection begins when the virus attaches to a cell and is able to enter it and use the cell's materials to reproduce. When that is recognized and nasal tests are done for the virus they show up as positive several days later when the results come back and the person is told to self quarantine for two weeks with no treatment.

This ignores both the pre-infection phase and the time when the virus is limited to the nose and has not spread. Looking first at the pre-infection period, we focus on our defenses as discussed throughout this book. These are respiratory infections and if, as seen earlier, the humidity in the air we breathe is greater than 50% they tend not to happen.

Looking specifically at where the virus enters the body, researchers from the University of North Carolina (UNC) showed how the nose is central in the infection and argued for its treatment there, but when a person tests positive—and ignoring the several days that a positive person can spread the virus before the test results are known—they are sent home to self quarantine with no treatment at all. At least this is the case since the president's preferred drug, hydroxychloroquine, was demonstrated in broad and controlled studies to cause more harm than good. These North Carolina researchers included one referenced earlier in this book who helped demonstrate the value of the sugar complexes on our nasal mucus and how they offer binding sites to infectious agents that prevent them from binding to us. Those complexes work on viruses too, but they are both natural and not patentable—read that as profitable, which is the bottom line in our current practice.

As argued throughout this book—and shown in Figure 7.1 on the next page—optimizing, optimizing our nasal defenses is easily done with the regular use of a xylitol spray that minimizes your risks before exposure to the virus. And it may operate by binding with the virus in the same way we have argued it binds with many bacteria. Unfortunately, there is no easy way to determine if this is the way it works except with broad clinical studies in people who use xylitol regularly. To restate our early argument: this interference method is preferred because it is soft power that persuades rather than hard power that kills. Hard power leads to resistance and continues our unwinnable war with microbes. Soft power persuades them to become friendlier.

Once the infection is established, persuasion is less practical. If the agent is the common flu, a nasal spray containing CPM is able to cope with the virus in the nose; furthermore, the spray has been used safely by nebulizer to deliver the virucidal elements to the lungs as well. The same holds for the virus behind the COVID-19 pandemic with the active agent being the GSE rather than the CPM.

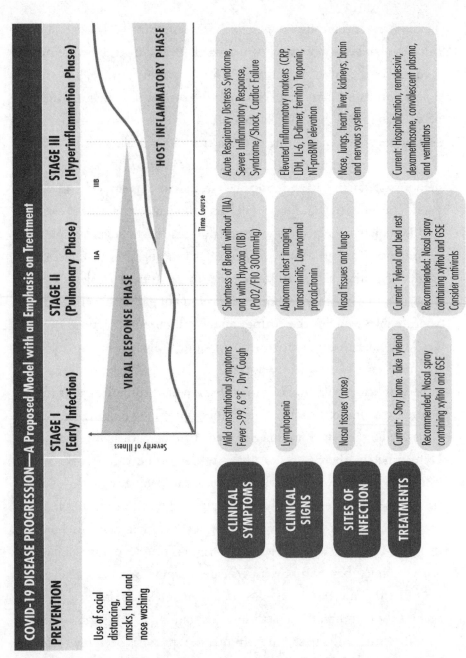

Adapted from Siddiqi, et. al. COVID-19 illness in native and immunosuppressed states: A clinical-therapeutic staging proposal. J Heart Lung Transplant, Vol 39, No 5 May 2020

Figure 7.1 *COVID-19 Disease Progression*

A significant benefit for both of these treatments is their direct application where the virus attacks. Oral delivery needs a much greater dose because only a fraction of it gets to the nose.

At the opening of this chapter I told the story of the cholera epidemic that led to the acceptance of oral rehydration by the CDC. At one of the several conferences on xylitol I was asked what would satisfy me that the message of xylitol had gotten out and my answer was that the CDC recommended it. That recommendation made little difference in our use of ORT in the US. My hope is that our pandemic will accomplish for the use of xylitol, GSE, and CPM what the Bangladesh cholera epidemic did for ORT. Dr. Ferrer and a hospital group in Florida are beginning a clinical study that will show how effective it is in coping with our current pandemic. Then it's up to the FDA. If the FDA demands more clinical studies because of the fact that there are no prior drugs using a nasal route to cope with a virus, then it's up to the alternative medical market. Drugs can make claims to help a medical condition, which is very useful if you have control over the drug and can get a patent on it. Absent that control anyone can step in and make the drug and profits needed to pay for the trials are not there. That's when alternative medicine steps in. In Bangladesh BRAC played that role.

For now, I would recommend to all persons who are medical personnel, first responders, or essential workers that they use the xylitol-saline-GSE nasal spray at least three- to six-times daily, washing their nose at the same time as they do their hands. That's what happened in Miami with Dr. Ferrer's COVID-19-infected colleagues and patients who used the CPM spray and were better in four days, and it's what happened in Bangladesh. We may well have a simple solution to the coronavirus. Xylitol-saline nasal products are widely available at drug and health-food stores nationwide.

As the *Good Men Project* noted in an article discussing our ongoing research, "The coronavirus appears mighty and powerful, but its nemesis could well be sitting in our medicine cabinet right now." Whether xylitol with GSE in a nasal spray will prove out in clinical trials isn't known; researchers need to watch carefully as they did in Bangladesh, but safety is not an issue. There is real hope that defense medicine will tame the SARS-CoV-2 virus.

CHAPTER EIGHT

Dental Health

I would be negligent if I wrote a book about xylitol and didn't touch on dental health, because that's where our story begins. I can promise you one more great benefit from using xylitol: far fewer cavities.

Unlike so many of our medical drugs today, where almost all side effects are bad news, xylitol offers some terrific overall health benefits.

This story begins in Finland with a few dental researchers. Knowing that sugar in our diets promoted decay they asked: What would happen if we used alternate sweeteners? The first study they did to check this out looked at the change in the amount of decay over a two-year test period in a number of people. The people were divided into three groups: one group used regular sugar to sweeten their diets, another used fructose, and a third used xylitol. The amount of tooth decay was measured before and after. Those that ate regular sugar had the most decay. Those that ate fructose had less, but those eating xylitol had none. This was the first of the "Turku Sugar Studies."

In Finland, where the government provides health services, this was good news because prevention is almost always better and less expensive than treatment. But internationally approved drug laws still handicap the government from allowing the drug claims that xylitol prevents tooth decay, so again, relatively few people know. Fortunately the size of this first study was such that the people in Finland were aware of it, and they did something about it. When you go to a dentist in Finland you don't get a toothbrush, you get gum.

After some further confirming studies the Finns started putting xylitol in chewing gum. Chewing gum is an excellent way to get xylitol to the teeth and an easy way to study dosing effects (the overwhelming majority of the studies done since the 1970s have used gum). More than thirty years of such studies have shown that chewing two sticks of gum two or three times a day doesn't help much, but four times a day helps noticeably, and five times a day prevents about 80-percent of tooth decay. There is so much evidence for this that they began giving it to school children five times a day, which is how Dr. Uhari found out what it did for chronic otitis, and we got involved.

Researchers have conducted laboratory and clinical studies to find out how xylitol protects our teeth. These studies were also among the first to find out how tooth decay actually begins. First of all we have bacteria that live in our mouths and on our teeth. They make up the plaque on our teeth that the dental hygienist removes regularly when we have our teeth cleaned. This plaque is a biofilm, a home for these bacteria. Most of them are nice to us in that they don't infect us, but these researchers found that when many of the bacteria eat the sugars in our diets, they make an acid that eats through the hard enamel surfaces of our teeth. This is how cavities begin. The particular bacteria that do the most damage are called *Streptococcus mutans*. Studies on the preventive effects of xylitol have shown several significant effects of xylitol on this family of bacteria.

First, the researchers found that these bacteria eat xylitol thinking they can use it for food. But the bacteria lack the enzymes needed to digest five carbon sugars so they get indigestion; and not just simple indigestion.

When observed the bacterial structure is really distorted after they eat xylitol—it looks like they are literally writhing in agony. They also found that the bacteria did learn not to eat the xylitol. Fortunately for us and our tooth decay, when they learned this they also learned not to make the acid any more. Remember the message of xylitol to the bacteria: to "shape up or ship out?" This is an example of bacteria shaping up.

Other dental researchers have looked at what xylitol does to the biofilm on our teeth. Studies done in France showed that xylitol impaired the ability of many cavity-causing bacteria to both make biofilm and the acid.

LONG-TERM PROTECTION

One of the more interesting dental studies with xylitol looked at young children in Belize. This study was in two parts. The first part lasted two years and tested a variety of combinations of sugar alcohols in the gums.

Sugar alcohols all work to replace the glucose or corn syrup in our diets, and if the replacing of glucose and corn syrup was the reason for the benefit, they would all work equally well at reducing tooth decay. This and most of the other studies gave a significant edge to xylitol. There were no real surprises in the first part of this study with the xylitol-only gum performing significantly better than the other options.

The second part of the study was a follow-up, done five years later. During the interim the people received with no exposure to xylitol. Just as they did with all other studies, dentists looked at the children's teeth and counted the cavities before and after, comparing numbers in both cases. The results were surprising. As expected there was some decay, but they also found that the permanent teeth, which had erupted in the xylitol-only group during the first two yearlong study, had 95 percent less decay than the other teeth.

These children received a long-term benefit from chewing xylitol sweetened gum for two years. As we saw earlier long-term benefits are when a particular action leads to a benefit long after the action is finished. In a case involving a bacterial action such as tooth decay, long-term benefits are explained only by the bacteria either going away or changing their nature. The most reasonable guess for the particular benefit of the children in Belize is that the regular presence of xylitol while their permanent teeth were coming in led to a biofilm on those particular teeth that did not have any acid-making bacteria.

This is also the most likely reason for the benefits seen in the studies of children whose mothers chew xylitol gum regularly. Dr. Eva Söderling and her group in at the University of Turku, Finland, performed studies on these individuals. These children were never exposed to xylitol, but they had significantly fewer cavities at age five than comparable children whose mothers did not chew xylitol gum. This benefit, like that of the children in Belize, likely comes from the fact that the biofilm on these children's teeth came from their mother's who used the xylitol regularly and did not have the cavity causing bacteria.

In Belize they were prevented because the children were chewing xylitol gum. In Dr. Söderling's group they were prevented because the mothers' chewing of the gum spread helpful bacteria to their children.

NON-ACID ENVIRONMENT

The eruption time for teeth is critical for the proper development of tooth enamel. As new teeth emerge into the mouth, the enamel is somewhat soft and porous. A non-acidic environment with the proper minerals strengthens this new enamel. Conversely the enamel can be easily damaged by an acidic environment, which eats through the soft enamel and keeps the needed minerals away. It goes without saying, new teeth erupting into such an acidic environment are considered to be at higher risk for decay.

Xylitol can provide crucial benefits for newly erupting teeth. Proper xylitol use provides an ideal non-acidic environment, and xylitol acts as a carrier for calcium, which enhances the natural mineralization process.

This combination of xylitol properties enables the new enamel to be optimally mineralized and provides long-term resistance to tooth decay.

TIMING IS IMPORTANT

There is a brief "window of opportunity" for a lasting protective effect when new teeth emerge through gum tissue. Ideally xylitol use should begin before the new tooth shows up, thereby setting ideal conditions to welcome in the new arrival.

Ages 0 to 4

The best way to prepare for a life of perfect teeth is to start at the beginning. Baby teeth ("primary teeth") are extremely important for the proper development and positioning of the permanent adult teeth. Decay can progress very rapidly through the thin enamel of the primary teeth. Tooth decay at a young age can lead to serious infections, as well as esthetic and orthodontic problems. Fortunately, early tooth decay is almost entirely preventable. Current recommendations include limiting the frequency of sugar consumption, especially between meals and before bedtime. But these are weak and poor considering what we know about how xylitol works.

Mothers should use xylitol to prevent transmission of acid-making, decay-causing bacteria to their infants.

They should start several months before the infant is born in order to shed the harmful bacteria prior to the time they expose their infants to these germs. Infants should use it to insure a proper environment.

Companies have put xylitol in a gel form that goes in a pacifier.

Ages 5 to 12

The transition period between baby teeth and permanent teeth is the "mixed dentition" time. For most children this occurs between the ages of five and twelve. Some consider this time as "the cavity—prone years," when children can satisfy their own sweet tooth with abundant sugary products. Fortunately, because of the xylitol products we now have available, this high-risk period can now be regarded as "times of opportunity."

There are lots of xylitol based candies, mints, and gums that will satisfy the child's desire for sugar as well as help their teeth develop. There are also a lot of recipes for baked sweets that use xylitol. Xylitol at this time changes the eruption period to one of enhanced protection as demonstrated in the Belize study—95 percent less cavities in these erupted teeth.

GOAL

Our goal is to have healthy teeth with no decay and no fillings. We now have the added protection of xylitol as extra insurance at those times we need it most. With the help of xylitol, tooth eruption can now be regarded as a great opportunity to develop the best smile possible.

Here is the bottom line: Using xylitol in the form of mints, chewing gum and toothpaste can help:

► Reduce cavities by up to 80 percent

► Inhibit the ability of cavity-causing, plaque-forming bacteria to stick to teeth

► Reverse early cavity formation

PART OF AN OVERALL STRATEGY

The California Dental Association recommends patients consider xylitol "as part of an overall strategy for decay reduction" and adds that, "With xylitol use, the quality of the bacteria in the mouth changes and fewer and fewer decay-causing bacteria survive on tooth surfaces. Less plaque forms and the level of acids attacking the tooth surface is lowered."

The benefits of xylitol are slowly being recognized. Did you know your dental insurance plan may cover xylitol-based products? Oral xylitol is so effective some dental insurance plans provide members with discounts on products. See if such products are covered by your dental insurance plan, and if they aren't ask them why not. It is clear that using xylitol regularly is a very effective way of preventing tooth decay. The U.S. military has recognized these benefits and now puts xylitol-sweetened gum in the packaged meals used by all of our military when they are deployed or in the field, but few of them are told what the gum is for.

Catherine Hayes, of the Harvard Dental School, wrote a review article on the beneficial effects of xylitol and other sugar alcohols in preventing tooth decay in which she said:

"Furthermore, since the evidence suggests a strong caries protective effect of xylitol, it would be unethical to deprive subjects ofits potential benefits. Given that several of the criteria for causality are met, *it is concluded that xylitol can significantly decrease the incidence of dental caries* [emphasis added]."

It is good that the U.S. military has the ethics to make xylitol available; it is lamentable that they don't talk more about it.

As with the spray, this is not a drug so drug regulations don't apply. This means that one can put very little xylitol in the gum yet still splash it all over the label. Again, check the ingredients list; if xylitol is not the first or second listed ingredient look for another product.

It needs to be remembered that xylitol is not absorbed as well as other sugars so more of it stays in the GI tract where it holds onto water. More water in the GI tract means looser stools. The gum tastes good, but too much gives you diarrhea. This is a very individual problem and your body does seem to learn. Most Finns do not report any problems with xylitol and those using it regularly do increase their tolerance. The up side of this is that putting a teaspoon or two in your coffee is a very good way to keep one regular—and it does.

HOW TO USE XYLITOL MOST EFFECTIVELY TO PREVENT TOOTH DECAY

► Look for xylitol-sweetened products that encourage chewing or sucking to keep the xylitol in contact with your teeth. Important: The best items use xylitol as the principal sweetener.

► Studies show that consuming four to twelve grams of xylitol per day is very effective. So have a wide variety of xylitol products: chewing gum, mints, toothpaste, mouthwashes, sweeteners, and more.

► Remember, if used only occasionally or even as often as once a day, xylitol may not be effective, regardless of the amount. Use xylitol at least three, and preferably five times every day.

► It's easy to keep track of your xylitol intake. "All xylitol" mints and gums contain about one gram of xylitol in each piece. You could begin with as little as one piece four times a day for a total of four grams. It is not necessary to use more than fifteen grams per day as higher intakes yield diminishing dental benefits.

► Brush with xylitol toothpaste. Xylitol-based toothpastes should list xylitol as their first or second ingredient (after water). Some toothpaste brands provide both xylitol and fluoride. The two are complementary.

► After eating, clear your mouth out with water and then immediately use xylitol. Between meals, replace ordinary chewing gum and breath mints with xylitol-based products.

ORTHODONTIC BENEFITS

Before leaving the subject of dental benefits we need to say a word about the likelihood of significant orthodontic benefits. I spoke at a conference on xylitol in 2009. When I finished an orthodontist asked if my nasal use of xylitol would prevent one of the most common and severe problems that he sees in his practice.

He explained that infants and children who breathe through their mouths change the tension of the facial and jaw muscles so that the palate raises and the jaw narrows. I can attest to the frequency of this problem since there are enough examples of it in my own family.

Ear, nose, and throat doctors think that mouth formation is not a developmental problem, but that the children are born that way. I tend to agree with the dentists on this because the individuals I know with the problem had serious nasal congestion when they were toddlers. There are also dentists in both the UK and the US who teach the importance of nasal breathing in order to prevent these orthodontic problems, and they routinely rely on our nasal spray to help.

While the argument is still in its infancy, it just adds to the reasons for keeping your nose clean. This is one that leads to major expenses with orthodontics, but it is not nearly as important as keeping the nose open to benefit yourself by optimizing the defenses that are there. Mouth breathing bypasses nasal defenses as well as the conditioning effect of the nasal membranes in the air we breathe.

THE DOWN SIDES

We cannot leave this part of the xylitol story without mentioning its side effects and its danger. We call it the "Two-D" problem: dogs and diarrhea. We do this here because the dental uses of xylitol use much more of it than when it is sprayed in the nose, and it is only when used in these larger amounts that it is a problem. For example, when Joseph Zabner was looking at nebulized xylitol for kids with cystic fibrosis he did a safety study on beagle dogs and everything was fine. But if you were to give those dogs, weighing about 35 pounds, a teaspoon of xylitol it could kill them. Dogs' bodies recognize xylitol as sugar and release insulin. The result is the decrease in glucose levels that is often lethal. KEEP XYLITOL AWAY FROM YOUR DOGS.

The other D—diarrhea—is a normal side effect of many sugar alcohols. Sorbitol, the sugar alcohol of glucose, is one of the more common treatment for the constipation that bothers so many elderly people. It has this effect because it holds water in gut by its osmotic effect. Xylitol has this same effect early in its use but is not used like sorbitol because one does get used to it. People are different too in how long it takes to develop this tolerance. Nasal use has never been a problem, but play with its oral use until you develop some tolerance.

CHAPTER NINE

Health and Healing Protocols

One of the most interesting "side effects" of xylitol is that it offers so many "side benefits." I am going to give you my thoughts and quick prescriptions for xylitol, as well as some of these fabulous side benefits. Overall, your health will benefit when you put some xylitol into your diet.

I'll also tell you about additional nutritional strategies that might be helpful to support your health and healing progress. Please be sure to work with your own doctor as you incorporate these into your health program.

ACNE

Acne is a common problem in those years when hormones blossom. It comes from bacteria getting into the pores of the skin which are then blocked with the thick secretions. I have seen significant success dealing with this problem when xylitol is used regularly in skin cleaning. Here as in elsewhere it seems to effect the bacteria that cause most problems.

Put a tablespoon in 4 ounces of a liquid soap solution and use regularly. It may take a while for the xylitol to dissolve so shake it up before using. Alternatively, if you are a user of "Oxy-5" squeeze out as much of the liquid from the pads that you can and add a bit of xylitol to it. Wait until it dissolves then put the pads back in and let them absorb the mix.

ALLERGIES

One more story. We have a friend whose life was controlled by her allergies. We don't get to see her that often, but she has called and told how her life had changed. She hardly notices her allergy problem anymore. She related that her physician husband had also recently begun to use the spray. She commented that he was a lot like Naaman, the captain of the Syrian army who wouldn't go bathe seven times in the river Jordan, as Elisha recommended in order to cure his leprosy, because it was too simple. Simple it is—keep your nose clean.

ASTHMA

A few years ago our doorbell rang. It was our postal lady. She had delivered our mail for some time and finally got up enough nerve to ask us if we were the people who had developed the nasal spray her husband had been using. We told her we were the guilty party and she thanked us. Her husband had asthma, and for years their lives had been controlled by his illness. Since he began using the spray his asthma had disappeared, and they can now travel and do what they want without having to consider the asthma. She said, "We got our lives back!" And so can anyone who is dealing with the problems we have been talking about. I only say this to reinforce my one big idea, one that works: Again, the key is regular use of your nasal xylitol—four to five times daily—each time you wash your hands. It's that simple. Keep your nose clean.

AUTISM

Xylitol won't cure autism, but it might prevent it. Many parents report lots of ear infections prior to their children developing autism. We don't have enough early and regular users to see if reducing ear infections helps prevent autism but it is still a good recommendation.

There is also another aspect of autism we would like to support that is related. Derrick McFabe is a Canadian researcher who looks at a particular small protein—propionic acid (PA)—that is well known as a messenger molecule that excites the brain. Putting PA in the brains of rats brings on autistic behaviors. McFabe paints out the correspondence between the onset of autism and the use of food preservatives using this chemical. He also shows how our high sugar diet feeds the bacteria that make PA, and that you can counter these bacteria by feeding your GI bacteria more erythritol, a four carbon sugar alcohol that shares many properties with xylitol.

BRONCHITIS

Bronchitis is inflammation of the bronchi, the tubes that carry the air we breathe from the trachea into all of the different segments of the lungs. Almost always this is caused by bacteria or viruses that have first colonized the back of the nose and subsequently gone into our respiratory passages because the mucus is too dry and can't hold them well enough to expel them. Mouth breathing also bypasses nasal defenses and increases the risk of bronchitis. Maintaining optimum nasal defenses with your xylitol—sprayed four to five times daily—is the best and easiest way to prevent bronchitis.

If you wish to supplement xylitol cleansing with herbs, certainly ivy leaf supplements are excellent for helping to relax the bronchial passages. They are used throughout Europe for this purpose and can be useful.

CANDIDA

Researchers report in an article, entitled "The influence of dietary carbohydrates on in vitro adherence of four Candida species to human buccal epithelial cells," published in 2005 in *Microbial Ecology in Health and Disease* (17;3:156-162) that consumption of xylitol may help control oral infections of Candida yeast by interfering with their colonization. In contrast, galactose, glucose, and sucrose may increase proliferation, according to the same article.

Get rid of the high-fructose juices. Perhaps worst of all is a diet laced with high-fructose corn syrup as found in altogether too many kids' beverages and other types of junk food. For overall health, this is so important. Water, alkalized preferably, teas, and other non-sugar beverages are going to help improve your condition.

I recommend quality probiotic formulas. Probiotics are beneficial bacteria that help the body maintain its defenses, especially in the gut where three-quarters of your immune cells are manufactured.

CANCER PREVENTION

There is a mushroom, *Cordyceps militaris*, known to have anti-cancer properties for a wide variety of tumors, from melanoma and kidneys to the brain. In 2017 Japanese researchers found that the active part of this mushroom's extract was largely xylitol.

CAVITY PREVENTION

Preventing cavities is how xylitol began as a means of improving our health. Xylitol talks to our bacteria and tells them to "shape up or ship out."

► Bacteria living on our teeth make acid from the sugars we eat and cavities are born as that acid then eats into our tooth enamel.

▶ Xylitol tells the bacteria to go away and to stop making the acid—and they do both in the end.

I strongly recommend that you brush with a xylitol-based toothpaste, chew xylitol gums, use xylitol breath mints, and use it in your cooking. The only thing it doesn't do in baking is raise yeast.

CYSTIC FIBROSIS

Cystic fibrosis is a genetic condition that affects the defenses of the airway by hampering proper mucus production. The mucus of children with cystic fibrosis is thick and not very moveable. A xylitol nasal spray helps this process. Using xylitol in an aerosol for administration in a nebulizer to the entire bronchial and pulmonary field is the focus of the University of Iowa group as they pursue their patent on this use of xylitol.

Every child with this condition should use xylitol both nasally and by nebulizer several times a day.

CHEILITIS (ANGULAR CHEILITIS)

Angular cheilitis is a condition caused by a fungal infection in the corners of the lips that causes them to crack and bleed. It is more common in older people, especially those with dentures.

Chewing xylitol sweetened gum has been shown to help reduce this condition.

DIABETES

Diabetes rates are skyrocketing. I see many more pre-diabetics with a constellation of symptoms, which include: obesity, hypertension, high cholesterol and triglycerides, and other symptoms of heart disease.

Diabetes is the inability to deal adequately with glucose, the primary source of energy for most animals.

The problem is either the inability to produce insulin (Type 1 diabetes) or for insulin to be effective (Type 2 diabetes).

In both cases dietary xylitol may help. In fact, xylitol was originally used as a safe all-natural alternative to sugar among diabetics. But, again, because of its low profitability, xylitol has lost out to drugs. Some research on its uses with diabetes continues. A recent South African study with rats showed its regular use normalized standard markers for the disease.

Possessing approximately 40 percent less food energy, xylitol is absorbed more slowly than sugar and doesn't contribute to high blood sugar levels or the resulting hyperglycemia caused by insufficient insulin response. In this way, cooking and sweetening with xylitol makes sense.

Introducing xylitol should be done slowly so that the body can increase those enzyme systems and pathways that metabolize it rather than leaving it in the gut where it increases diarrhea. When you do get used to it you can use it as sugar; it has the same sweetness as sugar yet has a third fewer calories. Yet that is not all. Many people with Type 2 diabetes have found that a low glycemic diet helps them better deal with their condition. They rely on what has come to be known as the glycemic index, which measures how much a specific amount (usually 100 grams) of a specific food raises glucose levels. The purpose of this is to decrease the glucose load with which these people must deal. Critics point out that people don't eat single foods and that the index doesn't deal with combinations of foods as they are more often served, but any effort to decrease the challenge of glucose to these people is a benefit. The glycemic index of xylitol is a measly seven, meaning it hardly has any effect on blood glucose.

Again with juvenile Type 1 diabetes, xylitol is a wonderful addition to the diet as a sweetener. It can only be of benefit to any child coping with juvenile onset of diabetes.

EAR INFECTIONS (OTITIS MEDIA)

For ear infections, of course, you will want to give your child xylitol nasally five times a day, as a preventive and during any prescribed treatment courses. Pediatricians have been warned repeatedly to cut down on antibiotic use and more and more recommend xylitol as a means of taking a proactive approach. I hope that with publication of this book many more pediatricians will get their earache patients using xylitol. It would be so good for reducing our number of special education students and help us to avoid overuse of antibiotics and ventilation tubes. Remember, if your child goes to daycare or school, you will need the help of their daycare workers and teachers if they are not able to wash their noses with xylitol spray alone.

FLU

Influenza or the flu is best prevented with the regular use of xylitol. Whenever you travel during cold and flu season, be sure to wash your nose with xylitol. Do it every time you wash your hands. Keeping your nose flushed with xylitol and moisture will help to eliminate the threat at the source. Also do the same daily for work situations.

Xylitol should also be used if you contract the flu—try to avoid, unless critical, the use of antihistamines and decongestants. In the long run, these will compromise your immune defenses, especially in the nose. On the other hand, the use of nasal xylitol will help to improve the defenses and aid in recovery time.

GAS

Intestinal gas comes from the bacterial breakdown of what we eat. Eating xylitol decreases the material the bacteria eat and reduces gas. Chewing gums, eating mints, and baking with xylitol will all help with this problem. I recommend taking a probiotic regularly to help too.

HEART DISEASE

I was working in an ER some time ago when one of our nurses was brought in by ambulance in the middle of a heart attack. He had not worked in the ER for the past few days because he was home with a respiratory illness. We took prompt care of his heart and he survived, but this experience joggled other memories of an association between cardiac events and upper respiratory conditions. We touched on this when we commented on Dr. Mehmet Oz's discussion of the importance of nitric oxide and how it relaxes the blood vessels and the lungs. Relaxing these things reduces the burden on the heart. If opening your sinuses where nitric oxide is made and released can help then we should.

But there is another way that xylitol can be useful. Heart attacks are caused by fibrous plaques in our blood vessels that break off and clog up an artery that feeds the heart. This happens more often when the body is in a state of chronic inflammation—like it's trying to cope with a chronic infection somewhere. The most likely place for that chronic infection is in pockets around our teeth where food and bacteria commonly find homes as we get older. Doctors teaching these ideas stress the importance of regular use of xylitol to cope with these oral bacteria.

HYPOGLYCEMIA

Low blood sugar is a problem for many diabetics and even some normal people. It is caused by increases in insulin secretion that drop the glucose levels by enough that symptoms are produced. The reason that xylitol helps this condition is discussed above under "Diabetes."

IMMUNE HEALTH

Xylitol positively impacts the immune system and seems to awaken the body's white blood cells much like other positively acting long- and short-chain sugars (polysaccharides). In rats, xylitol has been found to increase the activity of the white blood cells called neutrophils that are involved in fighting off bacteria. A benefit has even been seen during sepsis or blood infection, according to a May 11, 2008 report from Marjo Renko and co-investigators in *BMC Microbiology* (8:45).

MASTOIDITIS AND MENINGITIS

Mastoiditis is an infection in the mastoid bones that are next to the middle ear. They generally begin by extension from the middle ear. If this infection is not recognized promptly and surgically drained, it commonly opens and drains into the brain causing meningitis or infection in the brain. Again these bacteria most commonly begin in the back of the nose. Even epidemic meningitis caused by the bacteria begins in the nose. Dealing with this specific problem is only on my wish list because the idea of washing these bacteria from the nose is too new to have any research looking at this benefit. So again washing your nose with xylitol would be really smart if meningitis infections occur in your environment and location.

Occasionally, we see clusters at universities and in communities.

OSTEOPOROSIS

Xylitol also appears to have potential for help with osteoporosis. Dietary xylitol prevents weakening of bones in biological models and improves bone density. Again, cooking with xylitol and using it as a sweetener just makes a lot of sense.

PREGNANT OR NURSING WOMEN

Xylitol is not only safe for pregnancy but its consumption is encouraged. Xylitol studies show that regular use significantly reduces the probability of transmitting the *Streptococcus mutans* bacteria, which is responsible for tooth decay, from mother to child during the first two years of life, resulting in fewer dental caries. Xylitol mints and chewing gum and even sweetening with xylitol are all recommended.

Xylitol has no known toxicity in humans, and people have consumed as much as 400 grams daily for long periods with no apparent ill effects. Women may safely use xylitol during pregnancy, just inform your doctor.

OBESITY

Calories play a part in most weight loss programs. If you have a sweet tooth, xylitol has the same sweetness as sugar but a third fewer calories.

NASAL POLYPS

Nasal polyps are almost always a response to local irritants. Removing those irritants should prevent them.

They are currently treated with either nasal steroids, which turn off the immune system so it doesn't recognize the irritants, or with surgery. I feel it is better to prevent them in the first place. When they are present, the concentration of xylitol in the spray we use is greater than that of the fluid in the polyp; regular and frequent use should shrink them. Removing the irritants by the regular cleaning removes the stimulus for their development in the first place.

PEDIATRIC FEBRILE SEIZURES

Febrile seizures are a major concern of parents but are not a medical problem. If one is certain that the seizure is only due to fever, the advice of my pediatrics professor is appropriate: "for heavens sake, don't just do something, stand there."

The problem is that there are many other causes of seizures and, while they all look the same, many of them need further workup. Febrile children less than six months of age do not have an adequately developed immune system and always should be taken to the doctor. Febrile children over six months should be supported and made comfortable. Remember that a fever is part of your inflammatory response and is there because it provides a survival benefit. Don't rush to treat it. (But do seek appropriate medical attention).

The association of aspirin-treated fevers due to viral infections and the subsequent development of Reyes Syndrome has switched the emphasis to using acetaminophen, but in the animal studies, any lowering of fever with drugs in these artificially infected animals meant that more of them died. Maintaining adequate fluid intake is the most critical part of treating a fever so oral rehydration is important to remember, but anything the child will drink should be used.

Whether or not a person becomes sick with an infection depends on the severity, amount of the infecting agent(s), and the defenses of the host. Using the concepts presented here we should be able to augment those defenses and reduce, if not eliminate, much of this problem.

PNEUMONIA

The respiratory syncytial virus picks especially on small children, and it can lead to pneumonia. A common problem following these infections is the development of asthma. Our grandchildren have regularly attended daycare for the past twelve years and have escaped numerous epidemics where many of the children have been infected with this virus. The only difference has been the regular use of the nasal spray. So for all kids,this is very smart preventive medicine.

SINUS INFECTIONS

Sinus infections are the adult counterpart to childhood ear infections. Back in the days before I went to medical school there were books published on coping with bleeding and blood clotting disorders of the newborn. Then someone discovered that giving the newborn a shot of vitamin K eliminated them. Now the books just gather dust. Sinus problems will have a similar fate if we will just keep our noses clean. Wash your nose four to five times daily for best results.

TINNITUS

Tinnitus is a constant ringing in the ears. It can be a side effect of taking some drugs, but more commonly results from recurrent ear infections that affect the middle ear. Again, keeping your nose clean reduces these infections and should reduce the tinnitus.

URINARY TRACT INFECTIONS

Chronic UTIs should be treated with mannose or cranberry juice extracts for long enough to trade out the GI bacteria that cause this problem. By all means, if you can identify a practice, such as bathing, that may contribute to their recurrence, try to adapt in a way that helps prevent the self infection (a notable cause). Use of xylitol as a sweetener and in baking should also help, as will brushing and using chewing gum.

VIRUSES

The use of xylitol is associated with reducing viral adherence; the washing is beneficial for reducing the viral load, and this helps the immune system deal with infection more effectively. See also Chapter Seven.

WOUNDS

Wounds usually heal without problems in a healthy population, but when a person has diabetes, or circulatory problems they become major problems. Wounds in diabetics feet generally led to amputation while back.

Hyperbaric oxygen help preserve many, feet and legs from being amputated; and since many died within a few years of being amputated, it has helped many. Randy Wolcott, a wound care physician in Lubbock, Texas, began experimenting with xylitol after we discussed its possible role in reducing biofilm adherence. Combining xylitol with lactoferrin he was able to increase the healing rate of certain wounds, like those of diabetics or people with poor circulation, from 65 percent to 77 percent.

YEAST INFECTIONS

When I first learned about xylitol, I went searching for it at my local health food store. The staff there had been recommending xylitol for ages as a treatment and preventive for yeast infections. These infections are common in people with too much glucose, and using xylitol helped them to reduce that load while still savoring the sweet taste. (See also "Candida.")

⌒

CHAPTER TEN

Putting it All Together

While upper airway problems are the most common reason for going to the doctor, they are certainly not the only problems we have. Additionally, our airway defenses are not the only ones we should be honoring and supporting.

Our bodies are living systems that adapt to the environments in which we live. Sometimes we change the environment to make us more comfortable and compromise our previously formed adaptations. This is certainly the case with our central heating and air conditioning and our nose's defenses.

Sociologists have looked at groups of healthy people and found that they share what Aaron Antonovsky, the Israeli American sociologist and academician whose work concerned the relationship between stress, health and well-being, calls a sense of coherence with their environment and their condition. Their environment is meaningful to them—it is not hostile. They have a greater sense of understanding their environment, and they feel that it is manageable. In other words, it's something they are comfortable playing with.

We can learn a lot here from the bacteria. When they are threatened, they adapt by developing resistance in order to survive. When they are not threatened, they adapt toward living with the current environment.

Infection survival is not an issue so they adapt toward diversity and cooperation. This is the kind of adaptation we want to promote, and we can do that by making the adapting agent more comfortable as they play with the elements in their environments. This work, and this book, is the result of chronic ear infections, but people can and do adapt to these problems.

My wife Jerry was discussing the problems of chronic ear infections with a very successful and intelligent woman recently. When Jerry explained to her that one of the long-term problems of chronic ear infections was frequent mispronunciation, tears welled in the lady's eyes. She whispered that she herself had that problem, and that even though she was successful and respected in her profession, it had handicapped her whole life because she didn't take advantage of the many opportunities she had to talk because of her own embarrassment.

The educational facilities that deal with these problems are now available in our special education programs, speech therapy, and classroom and teacher modifications. The problem is that children who require these services are often labeled slow learners, and that label is seen as a threat or preordained conclusion to the kids themselves and their caring parents. It often prompts a defensive response that leads to each side digging in their heels as they argue over how to treat the child. More often, these are children facing difficulties that can be rehabilitated. They are not slow, and labeling them so does no good at all. Of course, the best way to deal with these problems now is to prevent them.

Jerry, too, when she read about many of the residual problems of early ear infections (the preference for silence, tone deafness, problems with syllables, and the same problem with pronunciation that plagued the life of the lady mentioned before), realized that her childhood ear infections had also left their mark. Penicillin was not readily available in the war years when Jerry experienced her problems, so her father comforted her by blowing smoke in her ears, without realizing, of course, that the secondhand smoke he was blowing in her face was a likely cause of her problem. But we do adapt, and when the environment is a loving one with caring people blowing smoke in your ears to comfort you, those adaptations are more likely to be creative and pushing toward wholeness because we are more comfortable playing with the elements in our environment when they are not threatening us.

Such play is more productive when it is informed. It would be best if you could find a physician willing to work with you, but there is enough information out there that you can usually educate yourself as well as relying on your physician; and, as I like to say, you may have better luck with your local biologist. Dental hygienists are increasingly filling this role when it comes to keeping your teeth healthy, but there are few counterparts in the medical area.

Naturopathic physicians do this and recent additions to chiropractic education enable it to do so as well. If you can find someone in your community with this kind of education, build a relationship with them. Ask them if they have read this book and what they think of it.

The play needs to be informed. It should not be a response to pain or other perceived threats, which could lead to the use of drugs and/or alcohol. Threats or fear leads to responses that come from the midbrain; the part of the brain that Yale Medical School neuroscientist Dr. Paul MacLean called the "reptilian brain" because it first showed up in reptiles. But the responses of this part of the brain to danger are mostly limited to fight, flight, or freeze. In order to be creative solutions they need some input from the cortex, the part of the brain that makes us human.

Creative play comes, again, with a sense of coherence—the condition is meaningful, manageable, and understandable. The elements for this creative play come from food and other materials— herbs, nutritional and dietary supplements, homeopathic remedies, mind-body work, and others—usually covered under the category of alternative medicine. The tools for using them come from an understanding of our physiology.

By far the best advice I have ever seen dealing with the food we eat is from T. Colin Campbell's *The China Study*. In his book he reports the results of the largest study relating food and health that has ever been done, and he comes down hard with the conclusion that our diets are far better if they are based on plant foods that are minimally processed. I would also add to his information, though I do it more in principle than with any evidence, that the more variety and diversity one can get in their food the more likely they are to get the nutrients they need to be healthy. That is advice as well for the farmers that grow our food; monoculture is risky since it makes it so much easier for pests to eliminate the entire crop. Almost as revealing as Dr. Campbell's dietary recommendations is his recounting of the hassles he has had to go through with the American food industry in his talking about what he has determined to be a healthier way of eating in his broad and in depth study.

Read *The China Study* and play with your diet. Those dealing with food allergies point out that one needs to follow a diet for at least a week before one sees an effect. Sometimes it's faster. Jerry had juvenile rheumatoid arthritis when she was younger. She got markedly better when she went on a pro- longed fast. She played with her diet. And she is not alone; other people with arthritis have seen similar benefits. She also found that avoiding red meat helps with her persistent whole body aches; and found this out after only two or three days on a cleansing diet.

And critically important in our play with food is including a wide variety of fruits and vegetables, preferably organic.

The sense of coherence that Dr. Antonovsky sees as critical in moving toward increased health, and the ability to play creatively with the elements in our environments, means that with creative play even how things fit together is open to adaptation; the goal is living in harmony with nature more than we have done.

I hope that, from this book, tens of thousands of more children and adults alike will find that they can breathe easy and live lives free of allergies, asthma, sinus problems, middle ear infections, and so many other URIs that plague us, not by taking a heavy-handed approach with our biggest guns and artillery (drugs and surgery) but by taming our enemy, keeping them subdued, outsmarting them in the end with superior ideas and methods. I try to make things simple for my patients and for all of you who have come to this book out of frustration and even desperation for help. It really is simple. I just go back to those caring words from my mom so long ago: "Keep your nose clean."

RESOURCES

HOW TO FIND XYLITOL

Xylitol-based nasal sprays, gum, mints, toothpastes, mouthwashes, and sweeteners are available at drug and health food stores, natural pharmacies, dental and doctors' offices, retailers and from other health professionals.

More Information:

Xylitol.org	**Twitter.com/xlearinc**
Xlear.com	**Instagram.com/xlear**
Nasal-xylitol.com	**Instagram.com/spry**
Twitter.com/xylitolcure	**Facebook.com/xylitol.experts**
Twitter.com/xylitolinfo	**HealthyLivinGMagazine.us**

ORAL REHYDRATION Q & A

Question: Who should use it?

Answer: Anyone who needs to replace fluids or who needs a little extra fluid because of illness, such as the fever discussed above. Definitely people with gastrointestinal losses should use this; that is what it is designed for.

Whenever someone is ill an IV will usually make them feel better. This is an IV you can drink. Pregnant women with nausea and vomiting can usually tolerate this and it prevents the dehydration that is usually treated with an IV. Extra fluid is always helpful when one is dealing with infection—it helps the washing. I have even used this successfully with diabetics who are vomiting, but vomiting diabetics can have serious problems and should be in a hospital.

Question: Should anyone not use it?

Answer: People with heart disease can get too much fluid and develop what is called congestive heart failure. Oral rehydration is not a good idea for them. If a person has an ulcer that is perforating the wall of their stomach they will have a whole lot of pain and their stomach will be rigid. Putting anything in a stomach with holes is not wise.

Question: How is it made?

Answer: Combine the following ingredients:

► 1 quart water

► 3/4 teaspoon salt substitute (read the little print on the package, this should be mostly potassium chloride)

► 1/2 teaspoon baking soda

► 3 tablespoons white corn syrup try to find one that is not made with high-fructose corn syrup (Karo).

For other than babies this may be flavored with juice concentrate or unsweetened powdered drink mix such as Kool-Aid.

Important warning: measure the baking soda and salt substitute carefully to prevent imbalance problems.

Question: How should it be used?

Some people chug it, but this is not recommended. Best is to think of it as an IV and drink small amounts regularly. The journal *Pediatrics* (1984 Nov; 74(5 Pt 2):950-4) in an article by LS Book entitled "Vomiting and Diarrhea" recommends the following steps for infants that can easily be adapted upward for older people:

▶ **STEP 1:** Wait one hour after the last episode of vomiting.

▶ **STEP 2:** Give 1/2 oz. (15 cc) to an infant or 1 oz. (30 cc) to a child over one year old every 20 minutes for one to two hours. If an infant is being breast fed only two feedings of oral rehydration are all that is usually necessary.

▶ **STEP 3:** If vomiting does not recur, increase the amount gradually. The goal is to replace the fluids lost within six hours. If vomiting does return go back to step 1.

If you have gone through this cycle three times go to the doctor.

▶ **STEP 4:** Advance the diet and resume normal diet in 12 to 24 hours.

Pay attention to your body; don't force anything on it that doesn't feel right. When you are adequately hydrated your body will know.

Question: Why use this?

Answer: In this day when we can stop diarrhea with a pill and calm an upset stomach with a shot why should one go through the turmoil? The best answer is to trust your immune system and try to support it in what it feels is best for your body. Some people whose diarrhea is caused by bacteria become carriers of those harmful bacteria when their diarrhea is stopped with medication. Some children have died of infection when they were given medicine that stopped their diarrhea. Trust your body.

ENDNOTES

CHAPTER 1

Harold Magoun Jr, DO, FAAO, FCA, DO, ED (Hon). "More About the Use of OMT During Influenza Epidemics," published in The Journal of the American Osteopathic Association, October 2004,104;10: 406-407.

The initial study on oral rehydration is: Sack RB, Cassells J, Mitra R, et al. The use of oral replacement solutions in the treatment of cholera and other severe diarrheal disorders. Bull World Health Organ. 1970; 43(3): 351-60.

The Lancet editors speak of oral rehydration as one of the most significant medical advances of the 20th Century in: Water with sugar and salt. Lancet. 1978 Aug 5; 2(8083): 264.

Anna Meinild and her colleagues explained how oral rehydration works in: Meinild A, Klaerke DA, Loo DD, Wright EM, Zeuthen T. The human Na+- glucose co-transporter is a molecular water pump. J Physiol. 1998 Apr 1; 508(Pt 1): 15-21.

Its lamentable use in the United States is reported in: Reis EC, Goepp JG, Katz S, Santosham M. Barriers to the use of oral rehydration therapy. Pediatrics. 1994 May; 93(5): 708-11.

CHAPTER 2

The safety of xylitol when it is put into the airway was studied by the group at the University of Iowa: Durairaj L, Launspach J, Watt JL, et al. Safety assessment of inhaled xylitol in mice and healthy volunteers. Respir Res. 2004 Sep 16;5:13.

The metaphor of dendritic connections as pathways that become roads and highways as they are used more and myelinated comes from personal conversations (pillow talk) with Jerry Bozeman, an expert in this area of childhood development.

The two articles in Medical Hypotheses are: Why the Increases in Upper Respiratory Infections? (2001 Sep. 57(3):378-81); The next step in infectious disease: taming bacteria. (2003 Feb. 60(2):171-4).

Luotonen M, Uhari M, Aitola L, Lukkaroinen AM, Luotonen J, Uhari M, Korkeamaki RL. Recurrent otitis media during infancy and linguistic skills at the age of nine years. Pediatr Infect Dis J. 1996 Oct. 15(10): 854-8.

Bennett KE, Haggard MP, Silva PA, Stewart IA. Behaviour and developmental effects of otitis media with effusion into the teens.Arch Dis Child 2001 Aug. 85(2): 91-5.

The study showing that tubes do not help reverse hearing problems is: Lous J, Burton MJ, Felding JU, et al. Grommets (ventilation tubes) for hearing loss associated with otitis media with effusion in children. Cochrane Database Syst Rev. 2005 Jan 25; (1): CD001801.

The study showing the benefits of chewing gum for ear infections was: Uhari M., et al. Xylitol chewing gum in prevention of otitis media.British Medical Journal. 1996 Nov 9; 313(7066): 1180-84.

CHAPTER 3

The dominance of bacteria in the scale of living organisms is from: Stephen J. Gould ed. The Book of Life. W. W. Norton & Co. New York, London 2001; p 5. Se also his article on Planet of Bacteria, in the Washington Post Horizons section1996(344):H1.

Resa Aslan's book, How to Win A Cosmic War (Random House 2009), applies to our war on terrorism, but it is just as applicable to our war with bacteria and coronavirus. Bacteria and nation-states are at the extremes of living systems that are better seen and dealt with as complex adaptive systems, what we call CASYs in our book The Boids and the Bees, where this issue is better explained.

Starfield B. Is US health really the best in the world? JAMA. 2000 Jul 26;284(4): 483-5.

Schappert SM. Office visits for otitis media: United States, 1975-90. Adv Data. 1992 Sep 8; (214):1-19.

One article showing the differences in asthma between the developed world and Eastern European countries is: Priftanji A, Strachan D, Burr M, Sinamati J, Shkurti A, Grabocka E, Kaur B, Fitzpatrick S. Asthma and allergy in Albania and the UK. Lancet, 2001 Oct 27;358(9291):1426-7.

The CDC study of asthma prevalence is: Mannino DM, Homa DM, Pertowski CA, Ashizawa A, Nixon LL, Johnson CA, Ball LB, Jack E, Kang DS. Surveillance for asthma—United States, 1960-1995. MMWR CDC Surveill Summ. 1998 Apr 24; 47(1): 1-27. Data for our graph is taken from their Table 1.

Information about South Carolina asthma incidence: Crater DD, Heise S, Perzanowski M, Herbert R, Morse CG, Hulsey TC, Platts-Mills T. Asthma hospitalization trends in Charleston, South Carolina, 1956 to 1997: twenty-fold increase among black children during a 30-year period. Pediatrics 2001 Dec; 108(6): E97 Copeland AR. An assessment of lung weights in drowning cases. The Metro Dade County experience from 1978 to 1982. Am J Forensic Med Pathol. 1985 Dec;6(4):301-4.

Svensson C, Andersson M, Grieff L, Persson CG. Nasal mucosal endorgan hyperresponsiveness. American Journal of Rhinology, 1998, Jan-Feb; 12(1):37-43.

Chris Post leads the Pittsburg researchers in looking at the role of biofilm in otitis. Post JC. Direct evidence of bacterial biofilms in otitis media. Laryngoscope. 2001 Dec. 111[12]:2083-94.

The data on the agricultural use of antibiotics is taken from a monograph done by The Union of Concerned Scientists: Hogging It: Estimates of Antimicrobial Abuse in Livestock, by Margaret Mellon, Charles Benbrook, and Karen Lutz Benbrook, Union of Concerned Scientists, January 2001 (report available at http://www.ucsusa.org/).

The role of biofilms in middle-ear infections: Luanne Hall-Stoodley, Fen Ze Hu, Armin Gieseke, Laura Nistico, Duc Nguyen, Jay Hayes, Michael Forbes, David P. Greenberg, Bethany Dice, Amy Burrows, P. Ashley Wackym, Paul Stoodley, J. Christopher Post, Garth D. Ehrlich, and Joseph E. Kerschner. Direct Detection of Bacterial Biofilms on the Middle-Ear Mucosa of Children With Chronic Otitis Media." JAMA 2006 July 12; 296(2): 202—211. Their results are worth repeating: Of the 26 children undergoing tympanostomy tube placement, 13 (50%) had OME [otitis media with effusion], 20 (77%) had recurrent OM [otitis media], and 7 (27%) had both diagnoses; 27 of 52 (52%) of the ears had effusions, 24 of 24 effusions were PCR-positive for at least 1 OM pathogen, and 6 (22%) of 27 effusions were culture-positive for any pathogen. Mucosal biofilms were visualized by CLSM [confocal laser scanning microscopy] on 46 (92%) of 50 MEM [middle ear mucosa] specimens from children with OME and recurrent OM using generic and pathogen-specific probes. Biofilms were not observed on 8 control MEM specimens obtained from the patients undergoing cochlear implantation.

Rayner MG, Zhang Y, Gorry MC, Chen Y, Post JC, Ehrlich GD. Evidence of bacterial metabolic activity in culture-negative otitis media with effusion. JAMA. 1998 Jan 28;279(4):296-9.

The study from Turku, Finland showing participation and likely cooperation between both bacteria and viruses is: Ruohola A, Meurman O, Nikkari S, Skottman T, Salmi A, Waris M, Osterback R, Eerola E, Allander T, Niesters H, Heikkinen T, Ruuskanen O. Microbiology of acute otitis media in children with tympanostomy tubes: prevalences of bacteria and viruses. Clin Infect Dis. 2006 Dec 1;43(11):1417-22. Epub 2006 Oct 31.

Ammons MC, Ward LS, Fisher ST, Wolcott RD, James GA. In vitro susceptibility of established biofilms composed of a clinical wound isolate of Pseudomonas aeruginosa treated with lactoferrin and xylitol. Int J Antimicrob Agents, 2009 Mar;33(3):230-6. Epub 2008 Nov 1.

CHAPTER 4

Arundel AV, Sterling EM, Biggin JH, Sterling TD. Indirect health effects of relative humidity in indoor environments. Environ Health Perspect, 1986 Mar;65:351-61.

Edwards DA, Man JC, Brand P, Katstra JP, et al. Inhaling to mitigate bioaerosols. PNAS, Dec. 14, 2004, 101(50):17383-388.

Silber G, Proud D, Warner J, et al. In vivo release of inflammatory mediators by hyperosmolar solutions. Am Rev Respir Dis, 1988 Mar;137(3):606-12.

Kontiokari T, Uhari M, Koskela M. Anti-adhesive effects of xylitol on otopathogenic bacteria, J Antimicrob Chemother, 1998 May;41(5):563-5.

Nathan Sharon and Halina Lis, Carbohydrates in Cell Recognition, Scientific American, January 1993.

Ofek I, Goldhar J, Zafriri D, et al. Anti-Escherichia coli adhesion activity of cranberry and blueberry juices, NEJM, 1991 May 30;324(22):1599.

Zafriri D, Ofek I, Adar R, Pocino M, Sharon N, Inhibitory activity of cranberry juice on adherence of type 1 and type P fimbriated Escherichia coli to eucaryotic cells, Antimicrob Agents Chemother, 1989 Jan;33(1): 92-8.

Kontiokari T, Sundqvist K, Nuutinen M, Pokka T, Koskela M, Uhari M, Randomised trial of cranberry lingonberry juice and Lactobacillus GG drink for the prevention of urinary tract infections in women, BMJ 2001 Jun 30;322(7302):1571-76.

Naaber P, Lehto E, Salminen S, Mikelsaar M. Inhibition of adhesion of Clostridium difficile to Caco-2 cells. FEMS Immunol Med Microbiol 1996 Jul;14(4):205-9.

Akiyama H, Oono T, Huh WK, Yamasaki O, Ogawa S, Katsuyama M, Ichikawa H, Iwatsuki K. Actions of farnesol and xylitol against Staphylococcus aureus. Chemotherapy, 2002 Jul;48(3):122-8.

Durairaj L, Neelakantan S, Launspach J, Watt JL, Allaman MM, Kearney WR, Veng-Pedersen P, Zabner J. Bronchoscopic assessment of airway retention time of aerosolized xylitol. Respir Res, 2006 Feb 16;7:27

Zabner J, Seler MP, Launspach JL et al. The osmolyte xylitol reduces the salt concentration of airway surface fluid and may enhance bacterial killing. Proceedings of the National Academy of Sciences USA. 2000 Oct 10;97(21):11614-9.

CHAPTER 5

Profet M. The function of allergy: immunological defense against toxins. Q Rev Biol, 1991 Mar;66(1):23-62.

The asthma conference was the Keystone Symposium, which was held in Santa Fe, NM, February 2002.

Elliott MA, Sisson JH, Wyatt TA. Effects of cigarette smoke and alcohol on ciliated tracheal epithelium and inflammatory cell recruitment. Am J Respir Cell Mol Bio, 2007 Apr; 36(4):452-9.

Rogers DF. Airway goblet cells: responsive and adaptable front-line defenders. Europ Respiratory J, 1994, Sep; 7(9):1690-706.

CHAPTER 6

David Satcher, M.D., Ph.D. Emerging Infections: Getting Ahead of the Curve. Emerging Infectious Disease, Jan-Mar 1995; 1(1):1-6.

The Plexus Institute conference was Complexity Science, Healthcare and Nursing, was held in Standish, Maine from 12 to 14 July 2009.

Paul Ewald wrote The Evolution of Infectious Disease. Oxford University Press, 1994. The information on HIV/AIDS is introduced in this book, but confirmed and elaborated later in personal communications.

Joseph S. Nye Jr. Soft Power: The Means To Success In World Politics. Public Affairs Press, 2005.

Much useful information on the down side of antibiotics comes from Dr. J. Douglas Bremner of Emory University School of Medicine and his book: Before you Take that Pill. A wide variety of information is available at his web site of the same name: http://www.beforeyoutakethatpill.com.

On the role of friendly GI bacteria see David Mindell, Evolution in the Everyday World. Scientific American, Jan. 2009; 300[1]:82-89. Most appropriate is the section on metagenetics.

CHAPTER 7

Studies on xylitol's effects on viruses: Yin SY, Kim HJ, Kim HJ. Protective effect of dietary xylitol on influenza A virus infection. PLoS One, 2014 Jan 2;9(1):e84633. doi: 10.1371/journal.pone.0084633. eCollection 2014. See also: Xu ML, Wi GR, Kim HJ, Kim HJ.Ameliorating Effect of Dietary Xylitol on Human Respiratory Syncytial Virus (hRSV) Infection.Biol Pharm Bull. 2016;39(4):540-6. doi: 10.1248/bpb.b15-00773.Disclosure in accordance with the Federal Trade Commission regulation 16 CFR, Part 255: this post is sponsored by an advertiser.

Effects of CPM on viruses: Wei Xu, Shuai Xia, Jing Pu, Qian Wang, Peiyu Li, Lu Lu , Shibo Jiang The Antihistamine Drugs Carbinoxamine Maleate and Chlorpheniramine Maleate Exhibit Potent Antiviral Activity Against a Broad Spectrum of Influenza Viruses Front Microbiol 2018 Nov 6;9:2643. doi: 10.3389/fmicb.2018.02643. eCollection 2018.

Effects of GSE on viruses: Miyuki Komura, Mayuko Suzuki, Natthanan Sangsriratanakul, Mariko Ito, Satoru Takahashi, Md. Shahin Alam, Mizuki Ono, Chisato Daio, Dany Shoham, and Kazuaki Takehara Inhibitory effect of grapefruit seed extract (GSE) on avian pathogens J Vet Med Sci. 2019 Mar; 81(3): 466—472. Published online 2019 Feb 4. doi: 10.1292/jvms.18-0754 PMCID: PMC6451896 PMID: 30713281

The University of North Carolina study: Yixuan J. Hou,et al. SARS-CoV-2 Reverse Genetics Reveals a Variable Infection Gradient in the Respiratory Tract Cell. 2020 May 27 doi: 10.1016/j.cell.2020.05.042 [Epub ahead of print]PMCID: PMC7250779 PMID: 32526206

My article in Medical Hypotheses: A H Jones The Next Step in Infectious Disease: Taming Bacteria Med Hypotheses 2003 Feb;60(2):171-4. doi: 10.1016/s0306-9877(02)00352-3.

CHAPTER 8

The first of the Turku Sugar Studies is: Scheinin A, Makinen KK, YlitaloK. et al. Turku sugar studies. I. An intermediate report on the effect of sucrose, fructose and xylitol diets on the caries incidence in man. Acta Odontol Scand. 1974;32(6):383-412.

An excellent summary of the intervening research is found in: Peldyak J. Makinen KK. Xylitol for caries prevention. J Dent Hyg. 2002 Fall;76(4):276-85. The story of xylitol is also told by these authors and myself in a booklet,

Xylitol: A way to better health, Woodbridge Press, 2004, available through most health food stores.

Tapiainen T, Sormunen R, Kaijalainen T, et al. Ultrastructure of Streptococcus pneumoniae after exposure to xylitol. J Antimicrob Chemother. 2004 Jul;54(1):225-8. Epub 2004 Jun 9.

The study showing how the bacteria learn is: Trahan L., Bourgeau G., and Breton R., Emergence of multiple xylitol-resistant (fructose PTS-) mutants from human isolates of mutans streptococci during growth on dietary sugars in the presence of xylitol. J Dent Res. 1996 Nov;75(11):1892-1900.

The recent French study looking at dental biofilm is: Badet C, Furiga A, Thébaud N. Effect of xylitol on an in vitro model of oral biofilm. Oral Health Prev Dent. 2008;6(4):337-41.

The two studies done in Belize are: Mäkinen KK, Bennett CA, Hujoel PP, Isokangas PJ, Isotupa KP, Pape HR Jr, Mäkinen PL. Xylitol chewing gums and caries rates: a 40-month cohort study. J Dent Res. 1995 Dec;

74(12):1904-13; and Hujoel PP, Mäkinen KK, Bennett CA, Isotupa KP, Isokangas PJ, Allen P, Mäkinen PL.

The optimum time to initiate habitual xylitol gum-chewing for obtaining long-term caries prevention. J Dent Res. 1999 Mar; 78(3): 797-803.

Söderling E, Isokangas P,Pienihäkkinen K, Tenovuo J, Alanen P.Influence of maternal xylitol consumption on mother-child transmission of mutans streptococci: 6-year follow-up. Caries Res. 2001 May-Jun;35(3):173-7.

Hayes C. The effect of non-cariogenic sweeteners on the prevention of dental caries: a review of the evidence.J Dent Educ. 2001 Oct. 65(10):1106-9.

CHAPTER 9

An excellent overview of xylitol's benefits beyond dental health:

Krista Salli, Markus J. Lehtinen, Kirsti Tiihonen, and Arthur C. Ouwehand*
Xylitol's Health Benefits beyond Dental Health: A Comprehensive Review

Nutrients. 2019 Aug;11(8):1813. Published online 2019 Aug 6. doi: 10.3390/nu11081813 PMCID: PMC6723878 PMID: 31390800

Simons D, Brailsford SR, Kidd EA, Beighton D. The effect of medicated chewing gums on oral health in frail older people: a 1-year clinical trial. J Am Geriatr Soc.2002 Aug;50(8):1348-53.

The article that Prof. Hudson refers to is: Hudson VM. Rethinking cystic fibrosis pathology: the critical role of abnormal reduced glutathione (GSH) transport caused by CFTR mutation. Free Radic Biol Med. 2001 Jun 15;30(12):1440-61. See also her more recent contribution: Visca A, Bishop CT, Hilton SC, Hudson VM. Improvement in clinical markers in CF patients using a reduced glutathione regimen: an uncontrolled, obser vational study.J Cyst Fibros. 2008 Sep;7(5):433-6. Epub 2008 May 21.

The South African study on diabetic rats is: Chika Ifeanyi Chukwuma, Shahidul Islam. Xylitol Improves Anti-Oxidative Defense System in Serum, Liver, Heart, Kidney and Pancreas of Normal and Type 2 Diabetes Model of Rats Acta Pol Pharm. 2017 May;74(3):817-826.

CHAPTER 10

Antonovsky, Aaron. Unraveling the mystery of health: How people manage stress and stay well. Jossey-Bass. San Francisco, California: 1987.

Campbell, T. Colin. The China Study: The Most Comprehensive Study of Nutrition Ever Conducted and the Startling Implications for Diet, Weight Loss and Long-term Health. Benbella Books, 2006.

For more information on how the idea of adaptation plays out in our cur rent society see our book: Jones, A. H. with Jerry Bozeman. The Boids and the Bees: Guiding Adaptation to Improve our Health, Health Care, Schools, and Society. The Institute for the Study of Coherence and Emergence. 2009.

INDEX

ABOUT THE AUTHOR

D r. Lon Jones, D.O., was a clinical assistant professor of family medicine at Texas Tech University Medical School and practiced at the Hi-Plains Hospital in Hale Center, Texas. He is the inventor and, along with his wife Jerry Bozeman, the developer and patent holder of the xylitol-enhanced saline nasal wash/ spray sold throughout the world under the Xlear brand. Dr. "Lon," as he is referred to by his friends, is a sought-after public speaker on nondrug methods for preventing and reducing upper respiratory conditions. His websites include Xylitol.org and Commonsensemedicine.org. He firmly believes that with xylitol "we have something that can optimize our nasal defenses and help millions of people worldwide."

He has written on other subjects in:

► *The Boids and the Bees: Guiding Adaptation to Improve our Health, Healthcare, Schools, and Society*;

► On Defense Medicine in *"From Microbes to Models: How coping with Ear Infections led to a New Paradigm."* Chapter 3 in *Putting Systems and Complexity Sciences into Practice*. Ed. by Joachim Sturmberg.

► On promoting general health in *"Revisiting Salutogenesis"* in *Embracing Complexity in Health*. Ed J. Sturmberg.

► On how health applies to society in *Let's Make America Healthy Again*.